THE WEIGHT ESCAPE

THE
WEIGHT
ESCAPE

How to Stop Dieting and Start Living

Joseph Ciarrochi, PhD

Ann Bailey, MA

Russ Harris, MBBS

Shambhala
Boston & London
2014

Shambhala Publications, Inc.
Horticultural Hall
300 Massachusetts Avenue
Boston, Massachusetts 02115
www.shambhala.com

9 8 7 6 5 4 3 2 1

First Shambhala Edition
Printed in the United States of America

♾ This edition is printed on acid-free paper that meets
the American National Standards Institute Z39.48 Standard.
♻ This book is printed on 30% postconsumer recycled paper.
For more information please visit www.shambhala.com.

Distributed in the United States by Penguin Random House LLC
and in Canada by Random House of Canada Ltd

ISBN 978-1-61180-227-6

Library of Congress Control Number: 2014951727

For Grace, Vincent, Helen, Grahame, Grant and Jenn
—Ann Bailey and Joseph Ciarrochi

For my nephews and nieces: Grant, Laura, Ben, Jordan, Andrew, Lara and Anna —R.H.

CONTENTS

INTRODUCTION

THIS IS NOT A DIET BOOK

How many more diet books must we buy before we realize they are failing us? How many more years shall we repeat the cycle of dieting hard, losing weight, regaining it all . . . and then criticizing ourselves for having failed to keep it off? Is this what we want our lives to be about? Will yet another diet book solve our problems?

Diet information is everywhere—on the shelves of bookstores, magazine racks, TV advertisements, internet sites, and in the mouths of our family and friends. By now, we know what we should do. We should eat more fruit and vegetables, avoid excessive salt and reduce our consumption of sweetened drinks and high-calorie foods. We know that we should exercise more. Yet what we *know* and what we *do* are two different things. Over 60 percent of us are overweight. If it was as simple as knowing that we should "eat less and move more," wouldn't we have worked it out by now? There is something standing in between us and our diet and exercise goals. That something is called "psychology."

This is not a diet book. This is a book about bridging the psychological gap between what we want to do and what we actually do. The book does focus on health and diet, but it puts health and diet in perspective, as parts of your larger life. Ultimately, the book is designed to help you move toward a life that is meaningful and vital.

Most of us live our lives like they are going to go on forever, waiting for the day when we are "good enough" or "thin enough" and can give ourselves permission to start living. What if we don't have to wait till we reach the right weight to start fully living, now, in this moment?

"Living in the moment" can be one of the hardest things for humans to do. To illustrate abstract ideas like this one, this book includes many brief stories, some based on our own experiences and others on people we've worked with. As you read these stories, consider how they relate to you and your own struggles; the issues might not be identical, but there may be enough similarities to your own life for you to draw useful lessons from them. Here's one now . . .

Sandra's story: going to pieces

When Sandra was three, she had simple needs. She wanted to play and she wanted others to play with her. She wanted to be loved and cared for. She climbed trees and balanced on logs and loved playing soccer with her dad. She loved eating cheesecake, and hated mint ice cream. She didn't much care if she was naked, especially around the house, and she danced and sang a lot. She cried a lot, too. After all, many things didn't go her way. She was three years old, a complete, complex bundle of emotion, energy and movement. She was whole.

Today, at 31, she's still complete and whole, but she doesn't know it. She hates the way her body looks and she avoids the mirror. She feels her thighs rubbing together as she walks. "Why did I eat so much at lunch?" she asks herself angrily. Her sister tells her she really should "look after herself" and recommends a new diet book. Then Sandra turns on the TV and watches thin actors fall in love with other thin actors.

Alone, angry, wanting to find love, Sandra opens the diet book. "I'll be disciplined. I'm going to be thin if it kills me," she tells herself.

Two months later, Sandra is transformed. She has lost 26 pounds. "Wow, you look great," her sister says. "You know what? I have a friend who'd be just perfect for you." Sandra knows she should feel happy, but to her surprise, she feels angry instead. And confused. During the week, other people comment on how good she looks, but none of it makes her happy. Now, instead of being satisfied with her weight, she wonders, "What did they think of me before?"

Sandra stops losing weight. The excitement is over. The diet says she can't eat her favorite dessert (cheesecake) or other foods she loves (rice, sweet potatoes). The diet makes her hungry and irritable. And here's the hardest part: after losing all that weight, she's still lonely. Indeed, she feels even lonelier than before because now she knows everybody thought she was "fat" before the diet. The diet has made her life worse. "I'm tired of being a good girl," she says one night, and eats a piece of cheesecake. Over the next two weeks, she gradually discards the diet. She regains the weight. Then she puts on another 11 pounds.

Sandra sits in her armchair and watches a TV advertisement about exercise equipment that promises to "rip fat off your stomach" in just 15 minutes a day. Maybe, she thinks, this will be the answer.

ESCAPING THE WEIGHT TRAP

What makes us become so narrow in our focus that we lose sight of everything except our diet and weight? What happened to the rest of our life? And why do we keep returning to the fad diets and crazy exercise schemes when we know full well that *in the long term* they don't work?

The answer is simple: we're human. We all get stuck at times. We all become inflexible, lose touch with what we care about and act in self-defeating ways that ultimately increase our pain and suffering.

In this book, we'll discuss the unique aspects of human biology and culture that lead to this state of affairs. We'll show you how and why we get stuck in "the weight trap"—that destructive cycle of dieting and long-term weight gain. And we'll show you how to escape that trap—how to get yourself unstuck and create a rich, full and meaningful life. Losing weight will undoubtedly be a part of this new way of living, but not the whole of it; you can't approach weight loss effectively without considering your whole life.

After all, your stomach isn't some separate part of you. Nor are your thighs, or your buttocks. They're all aspects of one whole person—you!—a person who loves and feels lonely, gets stressed and feels relief, a bundle of opposites and paradoxes. There's much more to you than your weight or the shape of your body. You have far more complex needs than can be satisfied by simply reducing the size of your stomach.

This is exactly why fad diets so often fail: they focus only on what you put in your mouth. They tell you to eat this, not that. They act as if you're nothing more than an eating machine. If it were so simple, there'd be no weight problems. It wouldn't be *normal* to be overweight. And there wouldn't be a multibillion-dollar diet industry and 125,167 diet-related products for sale on Amazon. So, obviously, this raises the question . . .

WHAT'S DIFFERENT ABOUT *THE WEIGHT ESCAPE?*

The Weight Escape is a unique program for wellbeing and weight loss. It will show you why so many popular weight-loss beliefs are simply wrong. For example, do you think you need to have a "positive attitude" before you can start to lose weight? Do you think that you need to be tough on yourself to stay committed to goals? Do you think that the key to diet success is to forbid yourself certain foods and deprive yourself of the things you love eating? Do you think the main reason you fail at diets is because you lack motivation or discipline? Do you think that to lose weight you must eliminate your cravings and urges to eat? All of these common assumptions are wrong, and this book will show you why.

The Weight Escape is based on a revolutionary psychological approach to wellbeing and fulfillment called Acceptance and Commitment Therapy (ACT). ACT is best known for its effectiveness in dealing with clinical problems such as depression, anxiety and addiction—but numerous published studies show that it is also of great benefit in reducing stress, giving up smoking, increasing physical activity and, of course, losing weight.

ACT utilizes a wide range of experiential exercises to reduce the power of destructive mental, behavioral and emotional processes. However, it doesn't see these processes as "symptoms" that can be "cured." Rather ACT recognizes that they are a normal part of every human life. ACT helps people to become aware of and at peace with their difficult feelings and thoughts, to develop kindness toward themselves, to live in the present moment, and to take value-consistent action.

The ACT approach will not tell you to deny your desires in order to lose weight. It will never suggest that there is something wrong with you or that you need to be hard on yourself in order to succeed. It won't tell you that you need to "think positively" in order to achieve positive results. Rather, ACT will teach you how to engage in health-promoting behaviors, even when you are feeling negative emotions, cravings, or a lack of motivation. It will show you how to use mindfulness skills to let go of useless struggles with yourself and your body and to escape self-destructive mindsets. Most importantly, ACT will help you to clarify what it is you most care about in your life—in health and other domains—and show you how to get it.

(There is a large amount of scientific literature that attests to the effectiveness of ACT and its various applications. You can find more information at theweightescape.com.)

Many weight-loss programs succeed in the short term but fail in the long term because they don't deal adequately with the psychology of eating: the powerful psychological factors that readily trigger overeating and the strong emotional barriers to eating healthily.

This book offers psychological advice about weight loss. We haven't included too much concrete dietary advice because a lot of that is already available. We don't think you need yet another diet book, but we recognize that some people need guidance through the confusing array of diets. This is why, in Chapter 5, we list six scientifically supported principles for weight loss. These principles can be used with any healthy diet, whether it's high-protein, high-carbohydrate or vegetarian. The principles give you the flexibility to choose a diet that suits your tastes and lifestyle.

We believe the diet principles will be useful, but we don't expect that, on their own, they'll lead to weight loss. We all know there's a large gap between knowing what's good for us and actually doing it. We hope that this book, by focusing on psychology, will help you jump that gap.

Here are just some of the useful things included in this book:

- How to effectively handle urges, cravings, hunger, and difficult thoughts and feelings.
- How to motivate yourself in the face of setbacks and challenges.

- How to free yourself from a self-defeating mindset.
- How to take control of your actions so you can behave like the person you want to be.
- How to identify what you want most in life and set meaningful goals.
- How to overcome the common psychological barriers to healthy eating.
- How to get far more satisfaction from your food.
- How to use values and strengths to give your life direction, and make it richer and more rewarding.
- How to live fully in the present moment.

THREE CRAZY ASSUMPTIONS

This book is about you, the whole human being, not merely about your diet, stomach and thighs. It uses cutting-edge scientific principles not only to help you get fitter and lose weight, but also to help you connect with what you care about and find the strength and courage to create a complete life, rich in purpose and love.

We're going to begin with three crazy-sounding assumptions, which you probably won't accept at first. But we hope that when you've finished this book you'll have experienced the power of these assumptions:

1. There's nothing wrong with you.
2. You have everything you need to succeed.
3. You are whole and complete.

Your mind might be saying something like, "I knew I shouldn't have bought this new-age garbage!" or "Oh no! Are they going to tell me to think positively, or to 'love myself' or to practice positive affirmations?" If your mind is saying something like this, please don't close this book or set it on fire. We guarantee this book contains no new-age claptrap, no positive affirmations, no exhortations to "love yourself." It's based on a solid scientific approach and these three crazy-sounding assumptions will soon make perfect sense. So please, carry on reading and see where the journey takes you.

DOES DIETING WORK?

There are two extremes in the multibillion-dollar dieting industry. On one side, you have a group selling you products they say will help you lose weight "quickly" and "easily." On the other, you have a group selling you the idea that all diets are evil, that they never work, and that they even cause you to gain weight. The latter claims are reassuring if you're tired of dieting and want to give it up. And many people *do* want to give up dieting. The problem is, the anti-diet claims are not so reassuring if you genuinely want to lose weight. They make it sound impossible.

Fortunately, scientific research indicates that many people do lose weight and keep it off in the long term. Nobody can claim that all diets, everywhere, fail. If someone tells you this, they're probably trying to make you feel better but they're not giving you scientifically accurate information. Note, however, that we're not saying it's easy to diet. Nor are we saying you must go on a deprivation diet to be healthy. Indeed, the word "diet" has become such a loaded term that it's almost impossible to mention it without generating strong emotional reactions. So it's essential for us to specify what we mean here by "diet."

WHAT IS A HEALTHY DIET?

In this book, diet does not mean depriving yourself for eight to 12 weeks. Nor does it mean making radical, unhealthy, unsustainable changes to what you normally eat. Instead, when we use the word "diet," we're using it in the original meaning of the term: the food you tend to eat on an ongoing basis. Thus, unless we stop eating altogether, we're always on some sort of diet. It might be a high-fat, high-sugar, large-servings diet, or a low-fat, low-sugar, small-servings diet, or a vegan diet, or a junk food diet, or a high-protein, low-carb diet, or a Mediterranean diet, or one of 50,000 other types of diet. But the point is, as long as we're eating food, we have a diet. So the question we need to ask is simply this: does your current diet contribute positively to your health and wellbeing?

Let's further clarify that every single weight-loss program ever invented asks you to consciously make choices about a) what foods you eat, and b) how much of those foods you eat. (This is true even of those approaches that claim to be against dieting!) And *The Weight Escape* is no exception. Indeed, our main aim in this book is to increase your ability to choose consciously what and how much you eat in order to help you live the life you want.

THE CHOICE POINT MODEL

This entire book will be built around a simple model that is easy to remember and that you can use in your day-to-day life. Figure 1 shows you this model. The top of the model describes two possible paths we may take, at any given moment in our life when we are presented with a challenging situation. We may take the left-hand path and engage in behaviors that take us away from what we want. We often label these behaviors "bad habits." Alternatively, we can take the right-hand path, which takes us toward our goals. Unhelpful habits are most likely to occur when we are mindless, that is, when we are not paying attention to how we feel and how we are reacting. The key to breaking this habit is through mindfulness, or taking a mindful pause at the "choice point." This is the point in the center of the model, at the crossroads where we either move away from or toward what we want to achieve. We will use this model throughout the book to show you how both difficult experiences and our values and skills can impact upon our decisions, and also how practicing mindfulness will help us make conscious decisions to move us toward our goals.

A mindful pause at the choice point helps us to pay attention, on purpose, with curiosity, and to choose actions that take us toward a life we value. It helps us to disrupt bad habits and gives us a chance to build new, life-enhancing habits, rather than acting without consideration, which can lead us to compromise our values and lead us away from our wants. There are many ways to create a mindful pause, as this book will show you, but let's do a quick exercise now so that you can get a sense of what it is all about.

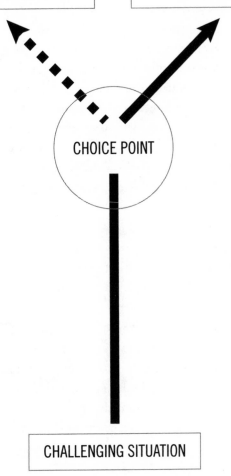

FIGURE 1: The Choice Point model

A mindful pause means S.T.O.P.

The simple acronym S.T.O.P. will help you remember how to create a mindful pause at important choice points.

S: SLOW DOWN

Slow your breath down. Breathe in slowly for 3 or 4 seconds, then pause, exhale completely for 3 or 4 seconds, and pause again. Do this a few times. Find a rhythm that is comfortable for you.

T: TAKE NOTE

Let your breath flow naturally now and just notice it. Notice each in-breath and outbreath as it comes and goes. Allow the breath to be exactly as it is. You do not need to do anything with it. Simply breathe and notice the breath and you will ground yourself in the present moment, where you are most able to discover and do what works. If you find yourself being distracted, acknowledge that this is completely normal. The mind is designed to wander. Gently bring yourself back to the breath and notice it.

O: OPEN UP

Make space for thoughts and feelings. Allow them to flow through you.

P: PURSUE VALUES

Ask yourself, "What kind of person do I want to be right now?"

Creating a mindful pause can help you change your life. It can allow you to acknowledge that negative emotions and thoughts are natural, while still empowering you to take actions that help you to fully enjoy your life and make positive choices in order to move you toward the things you truly care about; in other words, to act guided by your core values. The more we are able to pause and choose "toward" moves, the more our life will be full, rich and meaningful. This book will give you concrete skills that will help you to take a mindful pause at crucial choice points in your life (including those that don't necessarily have to do with weight loss).

Of course, it is not easy for us to live in the moment and make positive choices. All of us know what we "should" eat and "should" do to be physically fit, but so few of us are actually doing what we know is "good for us."

This book will explain why it is natural for humans to act in self-defeating ways that prevent them from achieving their long-term goals. Some authors refer to this as "self-sabotage," but we don't like this term, because "sabotage" is a deliberate, intentional act of destruction—and as we shall see, the vast majority of our self-defeating behavior is not deliberate or intentional. Rather, we do it automatically, or mindlessly, without really realizing what we are doing.

We will then guide you to weight loss through two major phases. First, after getting in touch with your own core values and formulating your weight-loss goals, you'll learn how to break free from self-defeating habits of mind. We all have these habitual patterns of thinking, and they often cause us unnecessary suffering and stop us from achieving our weight-loss goals. In Part 1 of this book, we'll show you how to break self-defeating habits, and rediscover your energy and freedom.

Once you've opened up space in your life, you can begin the second phase: building a rich and meaningful life. You'll learn how to overcome setbacks with self-compassion, how to shift your energy and attention toward the things you most care about, and how to develop empowering, life-enhancing habits. Part 2 of this book is all about recreating your life, habit by habit, until one day you wake up and find that your days are naturally filled with purpose and vitality. "Good" habits take the pressure off. They help us stay on track without always having to grit our teeth and rely on willpower to make healthy choices.

WEIGHT ESCAPE SUMMARIES

At the end of each chapter, you'll find a summary of the basic skills for weight loss outlined in that chapter. If you invest the time and effort to learn the psychological skills, you'll gradually find it easier to apply these principles to your life.

PART 1:

BREAKING FREE

I.

IDENTIFYING YOUR VALUES AND GOALS

Humans are both cursed and blessed with the knowledge that they'll die someday. We feel the urgency of time passing. We long to live life to the full. And yet how do most of us actually live our lives? We buy lots of things to make ourselves feel good, but we still feel dissatisfied with what we have. We socialize with many people—on the internet, at home, at work—but still feel lonely. We have access to every kind of pleasure—food, drink, movies, gambling, games, internet, music—and yet none of it is enough. None of it satisfies our longing for meaning and purpose.

We seek to satisfy our longing by buying more, socializing more and consuming more. We don't notice that trying to get more only makes us feel worse. Like drug addicts, we can't seem to stop. We sacrifice our time and energy in order to get the right house, the right qualification, the right job, the right car, the right clothes, the right "thing" that will finally make us feel like we have enough. When we finally have enough, we believe, we will arrive. But where?

We think there's something wrong with our body, and spend our time looking at ourselves in the mirror, trying to hide our flaws and wishing we were a different size. We refuse to go to certain public places like the beach or swimming pool because we feel too fat. We read book after book and article after article desperately trying to find the secret to weight loss. We sometimes get some perspective and wonder, "How many secrets could there possibly be?" and "How come these secrets never work for me?"

How many different ways can we be told to eat more fruit and vegetables, cut down on fat and sugar, and do more exercise? But still we search for the secret, still we cling to the hope that there's a quick fix, a simple and easy way to lose weight and keep it off. And many of us also believe that if we can just lose enough weight to get the look we're after, we'll be good enough. Then we can begin living life.

But life is beginning now. And now. And now. We're here now, and none of us will be here in 90 years or so. We're fellow travelers. How will we spend our time?

Ultimately, we each need to answer the same deep questions:

1. How will I develop friendship and love?
2. How will I positively influence the world?
3. How will I give and find joy?

In this chapter, we'll ask these questions again and again. And we'll encourage you to ask these questions of yourself as you read the rest of this book and for the rest of your life. You'll find that as you grow older and change, your answers to the questions will change, but the questions stay the same. The secret to becoming the author of your own life is not to have the right answers, but rather to remember to keep asking yourself these ultimate questions.

And here's something else that's important to remember: no matter what the magazines and popular books may claim, answering the next three questions won't deliver you a rich and meaningful life:

1. How do I lose weight?
2. How do I maintain weight loss?
3. How do I get the look I want?

Weight loss can never be an end in itself. After all, death is the ultimate weight-loss strategy. We want strategies for *living*, so it's important to remember that weight loss is only a means to an end. We do it in the service of a greater purpose. Ultimately, weight loss will be about improving our health—physical, psychological or emotional. Let's rephrase our ultimate questions:

1. How will weight loss improve my health?
2. How will improved health help me develop friendship and love?
3. How will improved health help me positively influence the world?
4. How will improved health help me give and find joy?

When we honestly answer those questions, we'll become motivated to lose weight and keep it off. And our life will be organized around a deep, guiding purpose. Weight loss will no longer be the center of our universe, it will just be a side issue, something we achieve as we go about living a meaningful life. We can make our life about something bigger than desperately trying to get smaller.

THE TWO HABITS OF UNHAPPY PEOPLE

See if you recognize either of these habits in yourself.

1. Striving to get away

The more we seek to avoid or get rid of our unpleasant thoughts, feelings and cravings, the stronger they tend to become. Furthermore, the attempt to escape these feelings drains us of energy we could be using to do something vital and authentic.

Suppose the idea of escaping our current weight and losing 20 pounds completely dominates us. That means that until we lose the weight, we'll feel inadequate. In other words, every day we're on the diet, we'll feel we're not good enough. Now let's say we succeed at the weight loss. "I'm okay now! I'm the right weight. Yippeeeee!" But then what? What will motivate us to maintain the weight loss?

Avoidance is a highly ineffective form of motivation in the long term. It often works for a short time, but eventually it sucks the life out of us. Sooner or later, we'll want something more. We'll look for something else to run toward. Authentic living often means moving toward something we care about rather than away from thoughts and feelings like guilt or not being good enough. We'll have much more to say about this soon. Take the one-minute quiz below to see whether you use dieting and exercise as a way to avoid unpleasant feelings.

ONE-MINUTE QUIZ: DO YOU DIET AND/OR EXERCISE TO AVOID DIFFICULT FEELINGS?

Do you think that dieting and exercising will solve your problems? Answer each question below as honestly as you can.

REASON FOR DIETING OR EXERCISING	HOW OFTEN DO YOU BELIEVE THIS REASON FOR DIETING OR EXERCISING?				
	NEVER	RARELY	SOMETIMES	OFTEN	ALWAYS
I do it to avoid feeling guilty.	0	1	2	3	4
I do it to avoid displeasing others.	0	1	2	3	4
I do it because of pressure from others.	0	1	2	3	4
I'd feel like a failure if I didn't diet or exercise.	0	1	2	3	4
I hate the way my body looks right now.	0	1	2	3	4
I don't want to be unhealthy.	0	1	2	3	4

If you answered 3 or more to most of these questions (i.e., you scored between 18 and 24), that suggests your health goals are primarily escape-oriented—that is, you're exercising or dieting mainly to avoid unpleasant thoughts and feelings. The truth is, we probably all exercise and diet to escape feeling guilty, at least a little bit. That's not a problem. It's a problem when our life is dominated by attempts to escape; when that happens, misery typically follows.

Karen's story: waiting for it all to begin

Karen searches across her bedroom floor, which is strewn with discarded outfits. She's stressed and rushing. Tonight she's meeting a guy she thinks she really might like and who might actually like her. But all her trusty outfits have become too tight. She can't get away with wearing any of them, but she has to, and she needs to hurry or she'll be late.

Karen feels her skin crawl underneath her clinging black pants. She feels disgusting and gross. Under the tension, she starts to feel tears sting her eyes. "No," she says, "don't cry, or your mascara will run and you'll look even more disgusting."

Karen has been trying to meet someone for years. Since her divorce, no one ever seems to work out. The best that ever happens is that she dates a guy for a few weeks, or at best months, and then he disappears. Lately, Karen can't even seem to get a second date. In Karen's eyes, there's only one reason she's divorced and alone: her weight.

A lifelong dieter, Karen has tried everything, and now she feels she's running out of time. She is 33 this year and really wants kids. She needs to meet someone. She needs to lose weight now.

Sitting in the bar, she waits for him to arrive. So far he's 20 minutes late. "That's okay," she tells herself. "The traffic is pretty bad." Twenty more minutes pass and she decides to text him to see where he is. No response. Fifteen more minutes pass. Nothing. She tries again, this time calling him. Voicemail. He's now officially one hour and 15 minutes late. It isn't going to happen. And here she is again; walking by herself to her car to drive home.

"I bet he took one look at my huge bum and ran away," she says to herself. She wants to call someone to talk about what's happened but she knows there's no point. Everyone's sick of her. They've heard it all before.

The only thing that keeps Karen holding on is the belief that one day a diet will work and she'll lose the weight for good. Only then, she believes, will she have a chance at the life she wants.

Most of the time, Karen wonders how she gets through the monotony of her days. One thing that really boosts her hope is hearing about a diet she hasn't tried yet. Karen jumps on board every new fad. Over the years, she's spent thousands of dollars on weight-loss "miracles." And she has had success, for a while, but the weight always returns. Still, Karen pushes on, believing that if she can just lose the weight, she'll finally be good enough for someone to want her.

Karen also believes that if she can stay fashionable, people will take her seriously. She subscribes to five fashion magazines. And every night, while the rest of the world sleeps, she shops online for new clothes, handbags and shoes. She loves the momentary high of each purchase, but the thrill never lasts. And now she has a room full of things she's never really used.

2. Building self-acceptance from the outside

Let's be honest. We all want to look attractive. If we want to lose weight, it's at least in part because we want others to like how we look. Striving to look good is not in itself a problem. But it readily becomes a problem when we *need* to look good on the outside in order to feel good about ourselves on the inside.

The biggest problem with building self-acceptance from the outside is that it simply doesn't make life richer and fuller. Research suggests that people who value attractive or prestigious things tend to be less happy and more antisocial. People who succeed at getting the look they've been after and hiding the signs of aging don't then feel good about their life; research says they actually feel worse. Of course, it's all about moderation. We're not suggesting you let yourself go—wear shabby, ill-fitting clothes and stop your personal grooming. We're merely saying that an excessive focus on your physical appearance, and trying too hard to make others find you attractive, is likely to make you feel worse in the long term.

The second problem with trying to feel good about yourself through focusing on your physical appearance is that it takes valuable time away from other things that are important in life. For example, consider Karen, who sought to build her self-esteem by shopping for things to make her feel attractive and glamorous. She felt excited when she was shopping and pleased right after she'd bought the stuff. But pretty soon all the new stuff is forgotten in the wardrobe. She must now work long hours to pay off her credit-card debt, which means she has less time to develop relationships or engage in other enjoyable activities.

Getting others to like how we look clearly doesn't bring fulfillment. We need to do something different. We need to find activities that give us a sense of joy and purpose. Once we have a clear focus for our life, we'll find it easier to commit to our health and weight-loss goals. Weight loss will become something we do for ourselves rather than to avoid unpleasant feelings or obtain the approval of others.

Take the one-minute quiz opposite to see if you waste time trying to feel good by focusing on your physical appearance.

ONE-MINUTE QUIZ: ARE YOU TRYING TO FEEL GOOD BY FOCUSING ON YOUR PHYSICAL APPEARANCE?

Do you care too much what other people think? Do you want to lose weight for yourself or to please someone else? Answer each question truthfully and take the opportunity to consider other possible ways you might try to feel good about yourself.

WAY TO BUILD SELF-ACCEPTANCE	HOW OFTEN DO YOU USE THIS WAY OF BUILDING SELF-ACCEPTANCE?				
	NEVER	RARELY	SOMETIMES	OFTEN	ALWAYS
I spend a lot of time trying to make myself look good.	0	1	2	3	4
I shop for clothes, jewelery and other things to feel better about myself.	0	1	2	3	4
I want people to admire my appearance.	0	1	2	3	4
I try hard to hide the signs of aging.	0	1	2	3	4
I feel envious of people who are thinner or more attractive than me.	0	1	2	3	4
I try hard to create an image that others will like.	0	1	2	3	4

If you tended to choose 3 or higher (i.e., you scored between 18 and 24), you're probably using a lot of your time and money trying to impress others, thinking that if they like you, you can accept yourself. We all do this to some extent, though, and even if you scored less than 18, this book will still help you avoid these kinds of behavior in the future and achieve your weight-loss goals.

DISCOVERING WHAT YOU CARE ABOUT

We all already know what activities *don't* deeply fulfill us, so let's now turn to what does. Ask yourself this question: what is important to you? Although it seems like a simple question, many people find it hard to come up with a substantial answer. However, if you take just 10 minutes to seriously consider it, it will help you to manage stressful events, improve your intellectual performance, improve your relationships with others and help you experience greater openness to life. And on top of that, it will also help you to reduce your weight and waistline. Hard to believe, right? Well, amazingly, research shows that all these things can be accomplished by the simple act of describing what you care about, or more technically, affirming your values.

Sound simple? It is! Yet how often do we do it? Let's try some value affirmation now.

EXERCISE: WHO AM I AND WHAT DO I CARE ABOUT?

The list below contains words related to values. Take some time now to look through this list and think about what's important to you. Then do the following:

1. Pick the three values (from either column) that are most important to you right now. Don't worry about getting this exactly right. You can always change your mind later. If you think of a value that's important but it's not on this list, just note it down instead.

2. Write a paragraph about why each of the three values is important to you.

Possible core values

- Connecting with nature
- Being curious
- Being fair or just
- Being loyal
- Being honest
- Being helpful
- Being sexually expressive
- Being genuine, friendly, open
- Being responsible, reliable
- Being ambitious, industrious
- Being competent, effective
- Protecting myself
- Being authoritative or in charge
- Being intimate
- Enjoying food and drink, and other physical pleasures in life
- Having a positive influence
- Being authentic
- Being self-sufficient
- Being analytical (e.g., solving problems, figuring things out)
- Self-development, self-awareness
- Learning
- Engaging fully, being mindful
- Caring for the planet
- Creating beauty

- Making a contribution
- Being courageous
- Being adventurous
- Seeking stimulating environments and activities
- Self-care: being active and fit
- Self-care: eating food that gives me sustained energy and health
- Being spiritual
- Being loving and caring
- Being respectful to elders and tradition
- Being self-disciplined
- Being appreciative of music, art and/or drama
- Being creative, innovative, inventive
- Being wise
- Resolving disputes
- Being constructive (e.g., building things)
- Being organized
- Engaging in clearly defined work
- Looking my best
- Being competitive (power)
- Caring for others
- Accepting (e.g., self, others, life)
- Being practical (e.g., working on practical tasks)
- Connecting with animals

USING YOUR VALUES TO CHOOSE YOUR GOALS AND ACTIVITIES

We've all spent time drifting. Like an unpiloted ship at sea, we've been pushed here and there by the forces around us. Sometimes we've tried too hard to please others. Sometimes we've rebelled, and done the opposite of what others wanted. Sometimes we've simply lost our way. No matter what we've done, we've always done something. Even giving up is doing something.

We're getting older and time is passing. We have no choice about that. But we *do* have some say over the direction we take. We can choose to guide our life according to other people's desires or our own short-term impulses. Or we can choose to guide our life based on our most deeply held values.

There are two major steps to making values the "compass" of your life:

1. State your values

What do you care about? Claim it for yourself. Values are entirely your choice. Nobody can tell you what you should or shouldn't value.

2. Experiment with values-based activities

Find concrete activities that put your values into play. See if you find those activities enjoyable and/or meaningful. If not, experiment with other activities.

Suppose, for example, that when you clarify your values, you realize you love being creative. Now you need to find a goal that supports that value. You may experiment with painting, but after doing this for a while, discover you don't actually enjoy it. You might then decide to experiment with a different form of creative expression, such as writing. It's quite normal for there to be a discrepancy between what we think we like doing and what we actually do. Values can guide us to certain activities, but only experience will teach us which of those activities is best for us.

Consider the value "self-care: being active and fit." There are literally hundreds of ways to put this value into play. We could go to the gym, take a regular walk or bike ride, or join a yoga class. It's usually impossible for us to use our mind to figure out what activity will be best for us. But it is possible to open our mind and let experience teach us what's best for us.

This brings us to a crucial distinction . . .

The difference between values and goals

Values describe how we'd like to behave in life, the qualities we'd like to bring to our ongoing behavior—such as to be loving, caring, kind, honest, open, engaged, appreciative, sensual, sexual, enthusiastic, disciplined or active. We can think of a value as a quality of action: a quality we want to model or embody in our behavior. We can use values as our compass. We can let them guide us as we travel through life.

Goals can be completed, achieved or ticked off a list as done whereas values can never be finished in this way. If your goal is to go for a 20-minute walk at lunchtime, you can achieve that: done! But if your value is self-care—taking care of yourself, looking after yourself—that value is never done; it's there for the rest of your life, until your final breath, and in each moment you can choose to act on it or not.

Here are a few examples of values, goals and desired outcomes and how they work together to build an enriching life:

Desired outcome: To be fit and healthy
Values: Self-care and self-development
Goal: Go to the gym at 6 a.m. this Monday

Desired outcome: A good relationship with my friend
Value: Being caring and loving
Goal: Help my friend move out of her apartment this Friday

Desired outcome: Enjoyment
Value: Being playful and creative
Goal: Engage in my hobby this Saturday morning

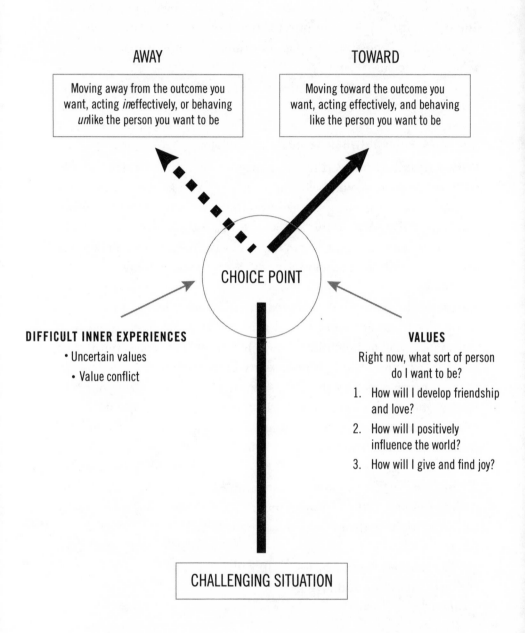

FIGURE 2: Identifying and affirming our values helps us move toward our goals

Another important difference between values and goals is that you can fail to achieve your goals but you can never permanently fail at your values. You could fail to go to the gym, for example, or fail to help someone or fail to engage in your hobby. But this wouldn't cancel out your values of self-care, being caring or being playful. The goals weren't achieved, true, but the values persist—and there are many, many ways, both great and small, you can still act on those values—today, tomorrow or a year from now. This is such a critical point that it bears repeating. *You can never permanently fail at your values; in each and every moment, you can either act on them or not.*

The figure opposite shows how our values help us move toward what we want. First we identify and affirm our values. For example, just before lunch, we might remind ourselves of our values, by saying, "My value is self-care. I want to eat healthy food because it makes me feel healthier and gives me sustained energy to do fun and challenging work during the day [value affirmation]. I commit to having a salad for lunch [goal]." Then, when we engage in the goal, we mindfully notice whether or not it serves our value. Did we in fact feel healthier and have more energy during the day? Sometimes we will discover that the goal does not serve the value. Perhaps the salad left us feeling fatigued, and we need to think about modifying our lunch plans somewhat? To use an example in the physical activity area, we may want to live the value "improving fitness" via the goal "riding a bike for an hour a day." However, after a week, we may discover that we hate riding a bike. That is when we need to consult our value again and choose a new exercise goal. If we keep reminding ourselves of our values, and experimenting with life, we will often find an activity that affirms our value and is also something we love or enjoy (or at least find easier to maintain than something we absolutely detest).

USING SETBACKS AS FUEL

In the health domain, it's natural to experience setbacks, but these setbacks only become a problem when they cause us to move away from our values. Say, for example, we gain 17 pounds over the holidays and are feeling miserable about it. It would be natural to say, "It's no use.

Self-care is obviously not one of my values. I obviously don't value taking care of myself." This conclusion is probably wrong. Your value of self-care is undoubtedly still there and there are millions of ways you can still act on it, even though you failed at this one particular goal.

Joseph Ciarrochi, one of the authors of this book, failed at his exercise goals repeatedly before he found an exercise routine that worked. He tried jogging for a few months, but eventually found it boring and painful on his knees and gave it up. He tried cycling, but found the roads to be too dangerous and unpleasant and stopped riding. He started working out at the gym during the workday, but found that he would often skip the gym, because he felt like "he did not have time." It was only after many life experiments that Joseph found the routine that worked: getting up at 5 a.m. every morning to exercise in the gym, before the demands of work could distract him.

Russ Harris, another of this book's authors, had the goal of writing a bestselling romantic comedy that would go on to be made into a Hollywood blockbuster. Alas, his novel sold only 2,500 copies and then disappeared from circulation. Goal not accomplished! Russ's values underlying that goal, however—being creative and entertaining others—still persist, and he's now writing another novel.

Ann Bailey, the book's other author, trained hard for several years in acting school only to enter the acting job market and find she could not get a job. After many months of tryouts and rejections, she realized she would have to do something else. Fortunately, there was a deeper value underlying that goal: a curiosity and fascination in why people do the things they do. Ann developed a successful career as a clinical psychologist, and was able to be curious about others from a different perspective. Now, Ann expresses her interest in others not by portraying a role on stage, but working closely with people and helping them to reach their potential.

The point is, no matter how many times we fail, we have the power to reassert our values. We have the power to say, "I didn't do what I wanted to do, but here I stand, and these are my values, so I'll try again." Fulfillment lies not in our ability always to remain firmly on the path of our choice, but in our ability to return to that path again and again.

HEALTH AS THE ULTIMATE DESIRED OUTCOME

Why do we think of health as an extra in our life, as something we'll get to once we've taken care of the "important things"? Why do we never seem to have time to exercise or shop for healthy foods and cook healthy meals? We're in such a rush that a multibillion-dollar industry has arisen to provide us with *fast* food. The supermarket is filled with highly processed unhealthy foods that can be prepared in just a few minutes.

But the major problem with putting our health second is that health underpins all our other values. If we're sick in bed or have little energy, we'll be less able to express friendship and love, influence the world and do things that are enjoyable. If we eat a diet that doesn't give us sustained energy, then sometimes we'll have a lot of energy, and other times we'll be tired and grumpy. And this moodiness may well push other people away from us.

At an intellectual level, we all know health is important, but all too often this knowledge does little to influence how we live. We frequently act as if our body and brain are self-maintaining machines that will never break down. This is because most of what goes on in our body is invisible. We can't see all those toxins and free radicals and hormones and biochemical processes we read about. We can't see the bacteria and viruses in our environment, or our immune system fighting them off. And we can't see when our body is nutrient-deficient and vulnerable to these pathogens. We don't notice when our body is becoming gradually but increasingly ineffective at processing sugar, a precursor to diabetes. We don't see our brain cells dying and our arteries clogging. When we hit middle age, we often don't notice the gradual loss of muscle mass with each passing year.

What we do see are the long-term consequences of unhealthy behavior: sickness, reduced cognitive function, decreased emotional wellbeing, reduced physical function and chronic disease. But do we really want to wait for these long-term consequences to happen before we change our life?

Let's return to our ultimate questions:

1. How will weight loss improve my health?
2. How will improved health help me develop friendship and love?

3. How will improved health help me positively influence the world?
4. How will improved health help me give and find joy?

To help you answer these questions for yourself, we encourage you to consider each of the nine benefits of a healthy diet and exercise below.

1. IMPROVED ABILITY TO THINK

Regular aerobic exercise is associated with better impulse control, faster processing speed and better memory. Increased consumption of fruit and vegetables is associated with better cognitive function.

2. IMPROVED ENERGY LEVELS

Low to moderate amounts of exercise increase feelings of energy and reduce feelings of fatigue. Low-GI foods—such as brown rice, cherries, spaghetti, whole wheat bread and some bran-based cereals—give you sustained energy over time (for more, see Chapter 5).

3. IMPROVED PHYSICAL FUNCTION

Exercise can be used to improve your strength, balance, agility and ability to play and do physical work. It also improves your quality of sleep. If you're overweight, a reduction of as little as 5 percent of your weight can reduce chronic physical pain and increase mobility, especially when you combine a healthy diet with exercise.

4. PROTECTION FROM ILLNESS

Exercise reduces the risk of developing coronary heart disease, stroke, diabetes and cancer. It lowers your blood pressure and plays an important role in weight management. Moderate levels of exercise are also associated with boosts in immunity. Fitness enthusiasts report fewer colds than their sedentary peers. About 40 minutes of brisk walking, five days a week, reduces sickness. Engaging in moderate to vigorous exercise reduces the chance of upper respiratory tract infections by 23 percent.

If you're overweight, modest drops in weight—about 5 to 10 pounds—can result in clinically significant reductions in blood pressure, and in the risk of type 2 diabetes and cardiovascular disease. Importantly, modest weight loss is associated with a lower risk of dying from any cause.

Probably one of the best things you can do to protect yourself from illness is increase your intake of fruit and vegetables. That will reduce your risk of heart disease, cancer and diabetes.

5. IMPROVED WELLBEING

Exercise reduces stress and its negative biological consequences. Research also suggests that on the days we exercise, we tend to have higher levels of life satisfaction than on days when we don't. If you're overweight, even small amounts of weight loss can improve your self-esteem and reduce depression. A recent study suggests that the more fruit and vegetables you eat, the happier you tend to be. The wellbeing benefit peaks at about seven portions of fruit and vegetables per day.

6. INCREASED OPPORTUNITIES TO SOCIALIZE AND HAVE FUN

There's no reason why exercising and healthy cooking have to be drudgery. If we're creative, we can make them fun. We can cook a healthy meal for our friends, for example, or take a cooking class to meet new people. Many forms of exercise take place in a social context, such as biking groups, cross-fit classes, team sports, and so on. We can sometimes make exercise more fun by turning it into a challenge. We can join competitions or just compete against ourselves, seeking to improve our speed or strength.

7. INCREASED SELF-DISCIPLINE

Self-control or willpower can be likened to a muscle. The more you work it, the stronger it gets. Those who exercise regularly, for example, demonstrate improved self-discipline in areas unrelated to exercise. Such people engage in more healthy eating, have improved emotional control, are better at monitoring their spending and have improved study habits. This means that if you pick one domain for staying self-disciplined, such as diet or exercise, you're likely to see benefits in other areas that require self-discipline.

8. SLOWED AGING

What would you do if we told you there was a fountain of youth but you'd have to walk 1,000 miles to get to it? You couldn't take any vehicle or ride any animal. Would you do it? If you did walk 1,000 miles, you'd be pretty angry when you discovered there was no fountain of youth at the end of the trip. But the walking would have done you a world of good. Just about any activity, including walking, washing the dishes and mowing the lawn, is associated with a lower risk of Alzheimer's disease. In addition to everyday exercises, resistance training is beneficial in preventing arteriosclerosis and age-related decline in muscle mass and bone density. Aerobic exercise, meanwhile, offsets age-related decline in the immune system.

Aging can bring a disturbing loss of muscle. We can lose more than 8 percent of our muscle between the ages of 40 and 50, and this loss accelerates to greater than 15 percent per decade after age 75. When we lose muscle, we lose not only our strength but our ability to function in the world. We struggle to lift boxes, play with our children, avoid falling, and climb the stairs. The good news is, much of this muscle decline can be offset with regular exercise. The images opposite nicely illustrate this point. They are cross sections through the human thigh. The dark gray is muscle, the light gray is fat (adipose tissue). Note how the thigh of an active 40-year-old and an active 70-year-old look similar, in terms of the amount of muscle. But notice how little muscle and how much fat there is in the thigh of an inactive 74-year-old.

40-YEAR-OLD TRIATHLETE

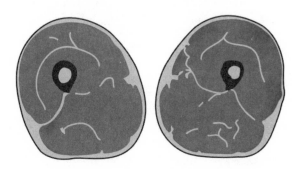

74-YEAR-OLD SEDENTARY MAN

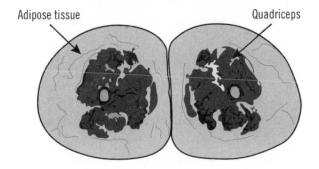

Adipose tissue

Quadriceps

70-YEAR-OLD TRIATHLETE

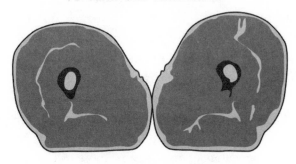

FIGURE 3: Intramuscular adipose tissue. The quadriceps of the active 40-year-old and 70-year-old look similar.

In many ways, fruit and vegetables *are* the fountain of youth. Increased intake of fruit and vegetables is associated with a decreased rate of arteriosclerosis, arthritis and cataracts. Increased vegetable intake is also associated with decreased age-related decline in cognitive function.

Unhealthy behaviors can accelerate the aging process. For example, being overweight in midlife and later life increases the risk of developing Alzheimer's disease. The more unhealthy behaviors you engage in, such as smoking, inactivity and low vegetable intake, the more likely you are to show age-related decline in memory and cognitive ability.

9. IMPROVED APPEARANCE

We live in a society that puts excessive emphasis on being thin and young. We will have much more to say about the damaging effects of these unobtainable ideals later in the book, but for now we wish to acknowledge that one reason we exercise and eat healthy food is to improve our appearance. We don't want to look like an anorexic (hopefully) but we do often want to look a bit leaner in our clothes. Exercise, healthy diet and weight loss can often help. The interesting thing is, if we exercise regularly, we can look leaner even if we don't lose weight. This is because a pound of muscle is smaller and smoother than a pound of fat. Imagine a baseball worth of muscle on your biceps. Now imagine a pile of jelly that has about 15 percent more size than the baseball and is crammed into your biceps. We're sure we would all prefer the size and look of the baseball than the jelly!

We have to be careful when we set appearance goals. We don't want to cling to them too tightly. The first eight benefits of diet and exercise listed above are almost exclusively for the self. "Improving appearance" is one of those activities that can be done for others. There is nothing wrong with wanting to make a positive impression on others, but we must always be aware that this goal has its dangers. We risk living so much for others that we lose our self. We can forget to care for ourselves and to live inside our own values. As humans, we probably can't help but worry about our appearance, but we can choose to hold our appearance goals lightly and not let them dominate our lives.

It is important to remember that the goal of "looking good" is itself always in the service of other values. If you want to look good in order to find a boyfriend, girlfriend, husband, wife or sex partner, then it's in the service of values such as love, intimacy, sexuality or sensuality. If you want to look good in order to have others treat you with respect or approval, then it's in the service of values such as respect or appreciation. If want to look good in order to stop criticizing yourself and start accepting yourself, then it's in the service of self-acceptance. If you want to look good because it helps you to influence others, then it's in the service of influence.

There are many different ways of serving all these values, without actually needing to look good. Please note, however, that we're not against looking good. We're not advising you to give up on it. We're just warning you that if you get too hung up on that particular goal and lose sight of all others, it's going to create more problems than it solves.

Matching your values to your health goals

Now that we've reviewed the benefits of healthy diet and exercise, it's time to connect our health behaviors to our most deeply held values. Use the values-clarification exercise below to develop your own health goals.

EXERCISE: CLARIFYING YOUR VALUES

Use the list on the following page to inspire and motivate yourself as you work through the rest of this book. Keeping your values and goals uppermost in your mind will help you get where you want to be. Explore what sort of person you want to be, then rate how important each area on the list is for you—from 0 (not important) to 10 (of the highest importance)—and the extent to which your health is related to that valued area.

VALUED AREA	EXAMPLE VALUES	WHAT SORT OF PERSON WOULD YOU LIKE TO BE IN THIS AREA?	IMPORTANCE (0 TO 10)	EFFECT OF HEALTH & FITNESS
HEALTH AND FITNESS	Engaging in exercise; playing sports; caring for myself; being active, being mobile; engaging in activities likely to give me greater strength, endurance, flexibility or energy; enhancing my appearance; managing stress			Not applicable
INTIMATE RELATIONSHIPS	Caring; supporting; connecting; accepting; being honest; opening up; nurturing; communicating well; helping; loving; being assertive, being attentive; being present; listening; having fun; being forgiving; being kind			
FRIENDSHIP AND OTHER RELATIONS	Same as for intimate relationships above			
PERSONAL DEVELOPMENT	Discovering; striving to understand; accomplishing; improving; learning			
WORK	Achieving; contributing; being effective; resolving disputes; having influence; building; creating			
SPIRITUALITY	Connecting with God or the universe; acting consistently with my religious beliefs or faith			
COMMUNITY	Promoting justice; caring for the weak; helping others; lending a hand; improving or protecting the environment			
RECREATION	Enjoying music, art and/or drama; listening to or playing music; creating; adventuring; discovering; collecting; building; enjoying food and drink; exploring; inventing; fixing			
SAFETY, SECURITY AND SUSTENANCE	Keeping myself and others safe from danger; providing for myself and others			

SUMMARY: IF YOU WISH TO LOSE WEIGHT . . .

DO MORE OF THIS	DO LESS OF THIS
Explore your values and remind yourself regularly what you care about.	Remain unclear about what you care about and what you want to do with your life.
Engage in activities that develop positive relationships, are challenging, are enjoyable and/or are important to you.	Engage in activities to escape feelings of guilt or because other people are pressuring you to do them.
Recognize that you can never fail at a value.	Believe that failing to achieve a goal (e.g., weight loss) cancels out your ability to choose a value (e.g., self-care). Give up.
Recognize how having good health will benefit all your values.	Fail to connect good health to your values.

2.
RECOVERING YOUR STRENGTH

Loch's story: a ticking time bomb

Loch is tired and angry. He didn't sleep last night. "Three years of work, designing this program and making it run smoothly, and they tell me it's not good enough. They tell me to improve it in the next week. It's impossible to do it that fast." He's walking quickly to the doctor's office, feeling the stress well up in his chest muscles. Lately he's been feeling this stress all the time. It's like there is a sniper in a tree, just waiting to pull the trigger. He has to keep moving or that bullet is going to catch him.

He stops and buys a doughnut. He's sweating from the heat. "When did it get so hard to walk?" he wonders.

"Borderline diabetes," the doctor says.

"Great," Loch thinks. "Something else to worry about. I don't have time for this shit."

Frantic exhaustion

We never seem to have time for ourselves. We run from task to task, our frantic days turning into frantic weeks and years. Our life seems to belong to other people. Even our bodies are not our own. Society demands that we look a certain way and dress a certain way and live up to impossible physical standards. So we do our best. We hand our time and fleeting energy over to other people. We work long hours, try to diet and exercise, try to be the perfect parent, partner, friend, worker, son or daughter—and still none of it seems to be enough.

If only we could get away. If only we could escape this pressure. Then we might start living, really living, the way we always hoped to live when we had those big dreams as a kid.

Loch in the story above has many forms of escape. His favorite escape is eating. When he's feeling stressed, he eats. He loves anything from the patisserie: doughnuts, macaroons, sweet cakes, tarts, cinnamon buns and croissants. Food is his drug of choice. Other people use chocolate. Not the cheap chocolate you buy at a gas station, but that really high-quality chocolate you can only get at some shops. Some people would swear that chocolate is better than sex (depending on who it's with!). These people eat chocolate because they love it, but also eat it when they feel lonely or bored or depressed.

Loch, like many of us, feels like he is always running from something. Maybe it's stress, or relentless pressure, or the feeling of not being good enough. Whatever this "thing" is, it feels like it's chasing him. He runs, but never fast enough to get away.

Food as energy and comfort

There's nothing more natural than to turn to food when we feel frantic and exhausted. Food is energy, and after a hard day when we're physically exhausted, food is what we need. But there's also emotional exhaustion, which takes many forms. Sometimes we feel sad and lacking in energy because life feels like a never-ending treadmill. We might give ourselves treats just to break up the tedium of the day. Other times we get no encouragement from the people around us. It's like nobody else notices when we do well. We might use food as a reward, as an apparent act of kindness toward ourselves.

Loneliness is common in our society, and comfort food can be one of the most potent short-term fixes. Think of all the occasions when food is used to nurture us and connect us with others. We get cake on our birthday or soup when we're sick. On those warm spring evenings, we might connect with our family and friends around a barbecue.

We might have an exciting night on the town with our friends, often starting with a restaurant, a few drinks and laughs. Major holidays like Christmas and Easter are often built around a feast. Food and love are so often connected that they almost seem like the same thing.

Escaping emotional pain

Food is just one form of escape. In this section, we're going to expand beyond food, because our life isn't merely about eating. We're going to look at our life as a whole, and all the ways we try to escape it. This is because we as humans all have something in common. We all have emotional pain and we all seek to escape it; this is as natural as removing your hand from a flame.

You may not believe that all people suffer the way you do. It certainly may not look that way. This is because humans suffer in secret. Our society encourages us to wear a smile no matter how we feel. If someone asks us "How are you?" we say "Good, thanks," "No worries" or "Can't complain." The most negative response we're allowed to give is "Not bad."

We definitely wouldn't say, "Well, actually I'm feeling really lonely" or "I feel like a complete loser" or "I've been thinking about running away from everything, just upping and going. It's all too hard!" We wouldn't say these things because people would look at us as if we were insane, or rapidly end the conversation and walk away. So we learn to hide our pain.

Fortunately, science allows us to look into people's hidden lives and see how much they really do suffer. Community surveys reveal that at any given time, one-third of the population will have a diagnosable psychological "disorder," and half of them will admit to being actively suicidal at some point in their life. People everywhere are struggling with divorce, anger at work, cancer, loneliness, financial stress, over-work, addiction, estrangement from their kids or parents, and more. Is there really anybody who's free from suffering?

And we all seek to escape. Of course, this also holds true for us, the authors of this book, and we'll make this point repeatedly by bringing in our own stories. We won't hide our struggles from you. After all, we're all, at some level, deeply similar. Here, for example, is a brief description of our author Joseph's struggle. Later in this chapter you'll find the stories of our other authors, Ann and Russ. We hope you recognize some of your own struggles in ours.

Joseph's great escape

My whole childhood I was led to believe there was something wrong with me. My father made me feel physically disgusting, like I was a disease-carrying bug. To this day, I remember him yelling at me for eating junk food and saying I was eating it because it was "sticky." I can still see the look of disgust on his face. I was a bug he wanted to smash.

I believed I was ugly. I had terrible acne, was considered too thin for a boy and was teased mercilessly at school. I wanted to hide myself in my room. I thought about suicide.

I carried my shame and insecurity with me into young adulthood, even after I left my father's house. I struggled to have relationships. Maybe, I thought, there was something really wrong with me and I didn't deserve love. Maybe I should give up. I sought escape in music and alcohol. I sought escape by reading book after book about World War II. I daydreamed about being a sports star. I was extremely poor and could only afford a single room in a bad neighborhood. I felt ashamed and I sought escape by telling myself I was brilliant and nobody could touch me.

Finally, I hit rock bottom and sought to reconnect with my father. We hadn't spoken for nearly a year, and I thought that if I could just reconnect, if I could just have a family, I would be okay. I knocked on his door. I can still remember him coming to the door, opening it, seeing me, then slowly shutting the door in my face and walking away. Soon after that I attempted suicide. Even that escape failed.

We need a pill!

Imagine we could design a pill just for you. That pill would let you escape any feeling or thought. What kind of pill would you like? Which of these feelings would you most like to make go away: stress, anger, frustration, sadness, fear, guilt, anxiety, shame, disgust, urges to eat, cravings for certain foods, hunger pangs, insecurity, self-loathing, fatigue, self-hatred, pressure?

Do you sometimes hate having these feelings? Do you sometimes want to push them away? How about these self-criticisms: not good enough, too fat, ugly, unlovable, unattractive, broken, flawed, weak, ungrateful, undisciplined, stupid, uncaring, selfish, loser? Would you like a pill to make those go away too?

We'll all differ in what we want our magic pill for, but we all want to get rid of something—some feeling, some self-criticism. Because we don't have a magic pill, we seek to control our feelings with other strategies. If we feel stressed, for example, we might try to control it by drinking, avoiding people, watching TV, and so on. Let's take a look at our author Ann's strategies.

Ann's great escape

Since I was a young child, I've always felt afraid. I've also felt afraid of my fear. I thought it would cripple me and leave me unable to live in the world, and do the things I wanted to do. I had to keep control of my fear so it wouldn't overpower me.

My parents signed me up for little athletics when I was seven years old. I was lukewarm about the idea until I discovered something. I felt good when I controlled my body and mastered it. It made my fear go away. When I was in this "controlling" place, I discovered I could finally feel still and safe. So the story began.

It wasn't that hard at first. I just had to keep moving (exercising) to keep the demons away. But eventually, when life got hard, staying in control of my feelings got hard. I often felt alone. I wondered why. I was constantly worried about what I said, what I did, how I looked, how I felt. Why didn't I have a boyfriend like all my friends? Why did the idea of intimacy terrify me? Why did I feel like such a freak?

I felt like I was living on a cliff face, waiting to fall off and disappear. I felt that my internal chaos needed to be controlled. And the only way I knew how was through my body. The more raw and helpless I felt, the more power and control I craved. So I ran and exercised and worried and beat myself into physical exhaustion until the day

I couldn't run any more. I broke down and it took two years of chronic illness for me to start to wonder why my life was nothing like I wanted it to be.

We all seek to escape ourselves

As you can see from our own stories, there are many ways we humans seek to escape from our feelings, to hide from the parts of ourselves we don't like. So our job now is to become aware of our escape strategies and their long-term effects on our wellbeing. If we make sense of these, we can begin to make wiser choices, and let go of strategies that ultimately drain our vitality and prevent us from flourishing.

EXERCISE: CONNECTING THE DOTSS

Grab a pen and paper, and answer each of the questions below as completely as possible. For this exercise to work, you'll need to be totally honest and think of the many strategies you use at one time or the other. You'll need to connect the DOTSS.

1. **Distraction**
   How do you distract yourself when you're feeling bad (TV, internet, computer games, magazines, music, etc.)? Do you ever use food as a distraction?

2. **Opting out**
   Do you ever avoid, withdraw, leave, give up, procrastinate or stay away from people, places, situations or activities that are important to you because you find them too stressful (in other words, you don't want to have the uncomfortable thoughts and feelings they cause)? Do you ever use dieting, eating or exercise as an excuse to opt out of other things? What do you opt out of? Social situations? Work? Doing things you love?

3. **Thinking**
   Do you ever try to think your way out of feeling bad? What sort of thinking strategies do you use (planning the next diet, problem-solving, worrying, blaming others for your problems, fighting with negative thoughts, wishing the past was different, fantasizing, daydreaming)?

4. **Substances and self-harm**

   Do you ever put substances into your body to push away unpleasant feelings (food, alcohol, cigarettes, chocolate, coffee, aspirin, acetaminophen, prescription medication, herbal remedies, recreational drugs)? Do you ever use food as a way to punish yourself? Do you ever harm yourself in other ways to dull emotional pain?

5. **Social strategies**

   Finally, what do you do in the social world when you feel insecure or upset? What social roles do you take on? When you feel threatened, do you play big? Do you play small and try to make yourself invisible? Do you become a bull, seeking to run down all discomfiting people? Do you play it cool? Do you play the clown or the joker? What sort of person do you sometimes pretend to be?

ANALYZING YOUR ANSWERS

Did you mention food as one of your strategies? We all eat to make ourselves feel better. We eat to comfort ourselves when we feel lonely. We eat because we're bored and want to feel stimulated. We eat to reduce stress or sadness. Sometimes we get angry when people tell us what we should eat, and so we eat to rebel against them.

The interesting thing is, we also *don't* eat to make ourselves feel better! We hate our bodies and go on an extreme diet to "punish" our body into shape. We believe the diet will finally give us the feelings we so seem to need: confidence, self-esteem and a sense of control.

We're not saying that *all* eating, dieting and exercise are about emotional control. Sometimes we eat for the pure joy of it, or simply because we need to in order to stay alive. Sometimes we diet because we have a deep commitment to health and vital living. Sometimes we exercise because it's fun and makes us feel healthy. What we're saying is that eating, diet and exercise are sometimes about control, about getting away from ourselves, and it's these times that can be the most problematic.

Whatever strategies you noted down for yourself, this book will help you to let go of them when they are making your life worse.

Is any of it working?

Now, take a good look at your strategies, like comfort eating and dieting. Almost all of them give you short-term relief from unpleasant thoughts and feelings, don't they? For example, we often feel good when eating our favorite dessert. But do any strategies *permanently* eliminate your insecurity, sadness, fear, self-loathing, depression, anxiety or loneliness? How long does your relief last before those thoughts and feelings return again?

If the emotion-control strategies worked, don't you think we as a society would be getting happier and happier? After all, since the 1950s, there has been an explosion of self-help books telling us how to get rid of or reframe negative thoughts. Yet there's no evidence whatsoever that we're getting happier. Our great-grandparents, who never read these "think positively" books, were probably just as happy as we are, if not more so.

It's not just self-help books that encourage us to control our feelings. Our entire society does. Do these phrases sound familiar to you?

- You've got to accentuate the positive, eliminate the negative.
- You don't want to worry about that.
- You need to take a positive attitude.
- You can beat this if you just stay positive.
- Don't worry, be happy.
- You just have to repeat positive affirmations and you'll be fine.
- Toughen up, princess.

Do we really think we can make all our suffering go away by repeating positive affirmations like "All my relationships are loving and harmonious"? Isn't it the case that we can still feel intensely lonely even when surrounded by people? That we can still feel hopeless, even when we have plenty of food and shelter? That we can still feel longing and emptiness even amid all the wonders of modern life? How much longer should we waste our energy on this futile struggle against ourselves? Does it not seem like our struggle against our feelings is taking us nowhere but away from what we care about? There's a different way.

Breaking the cycle

We have a choice about whether or not we want to end up like Sisyphus. Sisyphus knew he was having a bad day when he watched the god of death, Thanatos, preparing to bind him with chains and drag him down to the Underworld. Luckily, Sisyphus came up with a brilliant trick. "Hey, Thanatos," he said. "Those look like mighty strong chains. Why don't you demonstrate how they work?" Thanatos, not being the smartest of gods in Greek mythology, obliged by putting the chains on himself. Then, lo and behold, Sisyphus locked the chains in place, trapping Thanatos, and fled the scene.

The gods were angered by Sisyphus's trick. They caught him and condemned him to a terrible and hopeless task: to push a heavy boulder all the way up a steep hill. But just as he was pushing the boulder to the top of the hill, it proved too heavy and rolled back down. Sisyphus then had to go back down the hill and push the boulder all the way up again, but once again, just as he was about to reach the top, it rolled back down. The gods doomed Sisyphus to repeat this task for all eternity.

Our attempts to escape painful thoughts and feelings are like Sisyphus pushing his boulder up a hill. It's hard work, it takes all our energy, it's exhausting and it's never completed! We never seem to finally push the boulder over the hill. We seem to get so close. When we eat that chocolate or pizza, we definitely feel better for a little while. But sooner or later that emotional distress returns, just as the heavy rock rolls back down the hill.

We might feel that there's something wrong with us because we can't seem to get rid of these feelings permanently, but in fact no human can do this. And as long as we keep investing our time and energy in this pursuit, we're like Sisyphus, doomed to exhaustion and failure.

When "trying harder" is wasting our strength

Do you sometimes have thoughts like this: "I just have to control my urges and cravings. If I can't do that, then I'm just not trying hard enough"? How about this one: "I just don't have enough willpower"?

Our society teaches us that the harder we try at something, the more likely we are to succeed. Yet in this chapter we're suggesting the opposite, namely, that trying hard to control our feelings with food and diet doesn't work. Not convinced? That's okay. Here's a thought experiment that might help you consult your own experience.

EXERCISE: HOW YOUR MIND WORKS

Imagine we have a machine that can detect when you're thinking about chocolate cake. We hook you up to the machine so that you have electrodes on your head. Assume that this machine is 100 percent accurate and a loud alarm will go off every time you think about chocolate cake.

Now here's your task. While hooked up to this machine, we want you not to think about chocolate cake for one hour. That is, we want you to go one hour without setting the alarm off even once. And because we're worried you won't try hard enough, we're going to give you the most powerful motivation we can think of: we're going to point a gun at your head and threaten to shoot you if the alarm goes off even once. Could you be any more motivated than that? Are you ready to take the challenge? Don't think about chocolate cake!

How long would you survive before the alarm went off? Most of us wouldn't last a minute, let alone an hour. We'd be so pressured not to think about chocolate cake that we'd be checking constantly to see if we were thinking about it. And that would make us think about it.

What makes it particularly hard to not think about high-calorie food like cake is that it is everywhere in our environment. You probably can't drive more than 10 minutes from your house without seeing an advertisement for fast food. Everywhere you turn, there are cues telling us to eat. You see them on billboards and TV, and in grocery stores, gas stations, etc. No matter how hard we try, we can't seem to find a way to avoid thinking about food.

An exercise in futility

If this "try harder" mentality is wrong, then why do we continue to do it? Well, it turns out that sometimes trying harder does work, but only in the outside world. It's easy enough, for example, to figure out how to get rid of the rubbish in your front yard or remove ugly furniture from your house. Don't like the color of your bedroom? Repaint it. Don't like your car? Trade it in for a new one. Don't like your nosy neighbors? Move away to a new area or build a high fence around your garden.

The rule of the outside world is this: if you work hard, you can usually get rid of what you don't like. That's sensible, but what if this rule doesn't apply to the inside world of our thoughts and feelings? What if another rule exists for this world, one we rarely notice? The rule of the inner world states: if you don't like something in your inner world—that is, the world of your thoughts, feelings, memories, urges, and sensations— you usually *can't* get rid of it. Indeed, trying to get rid of it often makes things worse. The more important you make it to *not* crave chocolate, for example, the more likely you *will* crave it. The more important you make it to *not* have insecure thoughts about your body, the more likely you are to have them. Our feelings aren't like ugly furniture that we can remove whenever we want to.

Don't take our word for it about these rules. Look to your own experience. Is there something futile about trying to control your feelings? Have you succeeded in eliminating your cravings? Have you succeeded at knocking insecurity out of your mind, or does it come back at times? Haven't you had enough yet of wasting your energy on strategies that only produce more of the unpleasant thoughts and feelings you're trying to escape?

Here's our author Russ's story. See if any of it resonates with you.

Russ's great escape

I know from painful personal experience just how difficult life is when you're overweight, and how stressful and frustrating it is trying to lose weight. My weight issues started when I was about nine years old. I was a skinny little thing up to the age of seven, but by the time I was nine I was quite chubby, and by the time I was eleven many kids at my school liked to call me Fatso. In my later school years, my weight fluctuated, but I was always on the chubby side, and then, when I went to university to study medicine, my weight ballooned.

You might think medical students would be a compassionate and accepting bunch, but not all of them are. As it happened, many of my male "friends" thought it was great fun to tease me about my flab. I can recall one person in particular who loved to come up behind me in the corridors, grab my pot belly, wobble it up and down and say, "Whoa, look at that gut, you fat bastard!" One of my most humiliating experiences at medical school involved the "surface anatomy" classes, where male students were required to remove all clothes from the waist up, so we could practice examining each other's chest and abdomen. I was so embarrassed revealing my flabby body in front of all the students—male and female—in my group. And boy, was I relieved we didn't have to go below the waist!

I went through several periods at medical school where I followed fad diets and obsessive exercise regimes—and they worked, at least for a little while. I'd lose weight and tone up, and get myself looking trim and terrific, but it never lasted. I soon fell back into my old habits of living on junk food, eating piles of chocolate and avoiding exercise. And as the weight piled back on, my mind would beat me up, telling me I was fat, repulsive and weak-willed mercilessly.

By the time I graduated as a doctor of medicine, I was clinically obese. But that realization didn't stop me from overeating. Indeed, by the age of 25, not only was I heavier than ever before, I'd also developed high blood pressure. At this point in my life, I was practicing as a physician and on a daily basis I was telling my patients how important it was to exercise and eat well. Boy, did I feel like a hypocrite.

And yet, over the next three years, things changed. Bit by bit, I learned new psychological skills that had a profound impact on my behavior, and by the time I was 28, I dramatically improved my life. I'd found a way of managing my weight sensibly, keeping fit, enriching my life and boosting my general sense of wellbeing. I didn't know at that point about the psychological model used in this book (ACT), but I had fortuitously discovered many of its principles through other pathways. And while some "experts" claim you can't lose weight and keep it off in the long term, the fact is, I'm now 46 and I've managed to stay a healthy weight for more than 18 years. So clearly those experts don't know everything!

In all those years, the single most important lesson I've learned—not merely for a healthy weight, but also for healthy relationships, a healthy career and a healthy life—is the wisdom of dropping the struggle with discomfort. Whenever I forget this lesson (as I often do), and try once more to escape from my distress, my life gets worse and my suffering increases. You'd think by now I'd have learned this lesson, but I, like you, am a fallible human being and at times I forget everything we discuss in this book.

But the good news is we can all get better at remembering. And the more often we confront, with an attitude of genuine openness, the painful reality that escape and avoidance only make life worse, the more readily we can embrace an alternative approach—and begin to create a better life.

There is no problem to be solved

If trying harder to feel better isn't the solution to our suffering, then what is? Here's the stunning answer. The problem isn't that we can't find a solution. The problem is that we're looking for a solution. What if the following was true?

- You're not a problem to be solved.

Now read these sentences and notice how you react to them:

- You don't have to fight yourself any more.
- Your distress is not your enemy.
- Your hunger is not your enemy.
- Your insecurity is not your enemy.
- Your craving is not your enemy.
- Your loneliness is not your enemy.
- Your body is not your enemy.

What would happen if you stopped trying to battle your cravings, urges and impulses? Wouldn't you just lose control of your behavior? Would you start eating chocolate, pizza, or whatever your favorite foods are, and never stop? Would you eat and eat until there was nothing left to eat in the entire town or city, until you could no longer fit out the front door? We may be exaggerating a little, but these are common fears.

Basically, our fear of losing control causes us to push our feelings and urges away (just like Sisyphus and that boulder). But although it's perfectly natural to attempt this, we'll never succeed. We're pretty sure you know this already. After all, you've seen for yourself, many times, that control strategies like emotional eating can make the distress go away for a little while—but like the monster in a horror movie, it soon returns.

The alternative path: willingness

Are you ready to try an alternative strategy? Instead of trying to avoid your pain, are you open to discovering a new way of responding to it? This new strategy doesn't come naturally. It's something your culture didn't teach you, something that initially may sound rather weird or implausible.

We call this alternative strategy *willingness*, which means opening up and making space for our feelings, allowing them to flow freely through us, neither struggling with them nor getting swept away by them. Willingness sets us free; it opens up our energy and gives us back control of our actions so we can do more of what we really want to do in life.

Unwillingness is like being at war with ourselves. We invest all our time and energy in battling our inner demons: loneliness, fear, sadness and anger. We fight them until we're exhausted. We drink alcohol, watch TV, eat too much, diet too much, and stop doing what we love.

We can't win. But we have an alternative, which is to stop battling and make peace with those inner demons. They're part of us anyway. Willingness is like declaring peace on yourself. Are you ready for that? We know it's not going to be easy. You've been at war with yourself for so long that you've probably forgotten what it's like to be at peace. The chapters that follow will help you find that peace and discover freedom, choice and long-lasting commitment to your weight-loss goals.

ARE YOU WILLING?

We can summarize this whole chapter in terms of one question. We haven't been asking ourselves this question. We haven't even noticed that the question needs to be asked. But here it is: *am I willing to make room for my distress in order to do what really matters to me?*

Now there's a high chance you'll misunderstand what we mean by this question, so first let's clarify what we don't mean. By "make room" for it, we don't mean tolerate it, put up with it, grin and bear it, or grit your teeth and get on with it. Nor do we mean resign yourself to it, give in to it, or allow it to control you or overwhelm you. What we mean is, are you willing to learn a radically new way of responding to painful or difficult thoughts and feelings, a new way of handling them that's probably totally different from everything else you've tried? Instead of fighting against your distressful thoughts and feelings, or being swept away by them, you can open up and make room for them, and allow them to flow through you freely, to come and stay and go in their own good time.

So here's the question again: *am I willing to make room for my distress in order to do what really matters to me?*

There are only two answers to this question: yes or no. Sometimes we'll say, "No, I'm not willing to make room for distress. It's not worth the effort." At other times we'll say, "Yes, what's at stake here matters enough to me that I *am* willing to make room for this stuff, even though it's unpleasant." There's no right or wrong answer to this question, but one thing's for sure: life's full of challenges, and challenges bring distress. And the more often we say no to the challenges in our life, and to the distress that goes with them, the unhappier we'll be. Most of us would benefit from saying yes to more things. And in order to be able to say yes and mean it, most of us will need to learn a new skill: to open up and make room for distress.

In the following chapters, we'll show you how.

SUMMARY: IF YOU WISH TO LOSE WEIGHT . . .

DO MORE OF THIS	DO LESS OF THIS
Recognize that it's normal to have painful thoughts and feelings, and natural to want to get rid of them. All humans do this.	Hold onto ideas that you're weird or inadequate because you have distressing thoughts and feelings and you struggle with them.
Recognize when attempts to get rid of the painful feelings in your life become self-defeating or self-destructive.	Ignore, deny, or remain oblivious to your self-defeating attempts to avoid or escape distress.
Let go of trying to control how you feel when it doesn't work to make your life better. For example, if emotional eating doesn't make you feel better in the long run or help you control your life, let it go. If fad diets don't make your life better in the long run, let them go.	Continue to engage in unhelpful attempts to control how you feel. Use all your energy to get *more* of what you don't really want. For example, continue to engage in emotional eating and fad diets even though they make you feel worse about yourself and lead to more weight gain.

3.
FINDING YOUR TIPPING POINT

A tipping point is a "moment of critical mass, the threshold, the boiling point." It's the point at which a little push, a small event, can lead to dramatic change. We're now going to talk about how we can find these points in our lives.

By making small shifts in our behavior, we can set in motion a process that has the power to change everything for us. We can create tipping points in our life that move us toward what we love and care about rather than away from them.

Joseph's tipping point

When I was young, I used to exercise all the time. I don't know what happened, but at some point I just stopped exercising. I started spending my time in offices, bent over a computer, year after year, until one day I realized I was badly out of shape. My body didn't even feel like it belonged to me any more. It felt separate from me, like an old, rusty machine whose only purpose was to lug around my brain. My body was 20 pounds overweight. I ached when I moved it. I got tired from climbing stairs or playing with my children. How had this happened? I used to love being athletic, but now I just felt fat and old.

So I decided I wanted to lift weights again. The only problem was that I hadn't lifted anything for 22 years and was extremely weak.

As soon as I even thought about going to the gym, feelings of embarrassment and anxiety immediately showed up. I imagined all those muscle-bound guys hulking around while I'd be sitting there, straining to lift the tiny pink barbells in the corner, hoping nobody noticed me. On top of that, my mind kept telling me that with my hectic schedule I just didn't have enough time to add exercise to my life.

So I had to ask myself: *Am I willing to open up and make room for these difficult thoughts and feelings, in order to go to the gym?* This is a version of the willingness question we presented in Chapter 2.

THE WILLINGNESS SCALE AND FINDING YOUR TIPPING POINT

You might visualize the willingness question (*Am I willing to make room for my distress in order to do what really matters to me?*) as a scale. On the left-hand side you have unpleasant thoughts and feelings, or distress. On the right-hand side you have valued goals. You can see Joseph's willingness scale below in Figure 4. A scale like this is intensely personal. Only you can decide how things are weighted for you. In Joseph's case, he decided that the distress outweighed the goal. He said no to the gym.

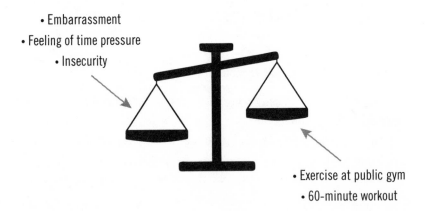

• Embarrassment
• Feeling of time pressure
• Insecurity

• Exercise at public gym
• 60-minute workout

FIGURE 4: Joseph's willingness scale. The distress (on the left) outweighs the value of the goal (on the right). Joseph avoids the gym to avoid distress.

The good news is that not only can we choose for or against a goal, but we can also choose the difficulty of the goal. If Joseph is unwilling to go to the gym for 60 minutes, then he can choose an easier goal. That is, he can find his *tipping point*, the point at which he goes from saying *no* to saying *yes*. He does this by choosing an easier goal and making the left-hand side of the scale lighter. In this case, he chose the easier goal of exercising in private (reducing his distress about exercising in public) and decided to exercise for only 15 minutes (reducing his distress at not having time). Then he asked himself again, *is the distress worth going for the goal?* And he ended up with the willingness scale below.

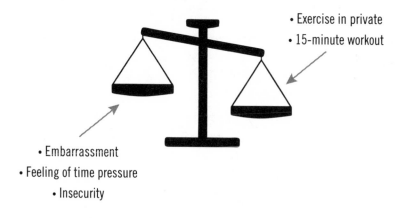

- Exercise in private
- 15-minute workout

- Embarrassment
- Feeling of time pressure
- Insecurity

FIGURE 5: Joseph's willingness scale, part 2. The value of the goal outweighs the distress. By exercising, Joseph makes space for the distress.

The willingness question is never permanently answered. Joseph might answer yes to exercise on one day and no on another. It's always a choice.

The interesting thing about our willingness tipping points is that once we start saying yes to something, even something very small, we start to behave differently. We start to make contact with the physical world and we discover new pleasures and sources of meaning. And when that happens, we want more. We're ready to start saying yes to many things.

Joseph's tipping point 2

Once I started working out in private for 15 minutes, I reconnected with the satisfaction of taking care of my body rather than neglecting it, and I especially appreciated how it lowered my stress levels, which in turn made it easier for me to be decent and generous to others (which is one of my core values). So by making the small choice to work out for 15 minutes, I discovered that I wanted to say yes again, but this time to a larger exercise goal.

My next step was to go to a public gym. To keep my insecurity to a minimum, I chose a gym that was open 24 hours. That way I could go at 5 a.m. and nobody would be there to see me lift the light, pink barbells. I also upped my workout from 15 minutes to 30, and began to see the gym as *my time*, as something of great importance to me rather than something that interfered with all the other activities I had to do as part of everyday living. My view of the gym had totally changed.

Sometimes things don't work out as planned. The first time I went at 5 a.m., I was shocked. I expected to find the gym empty. Instead, all of the Incredible Hulk–like construction workers were there! So now I was faced with the exact anxiety-provoking situation I'd sought so hard to avoid—lifting light weights in front of incredibly muscular guys.

I had to ask myself again, *is the goal worth the distress?* Do I go to the gym, even though it's more distressing than I'd originally thought? Or do I choose another goal? We all have to ask willingness questions like this again and again. On this particular occasion, I decided to keep going to the gym. At least I knew that none of the muscular men would fight me for the lightweight barbells.

Over time, I was surprised to discover that I actually loved working out, especially as it allowed me time to listen to audio books. I've now expanded my time at the gym from about one hour a week, to one hour on four or five days a week. My mood and energy levels have never been better. I may still be one of the weaker guys in the gym, and one of the older guys, but that stuff doesn't hold me back any more. I've now experienced the benefits of exercise and they simply overwhelm the distress.

LEARNING TO SAY YES

Joseph's story is inspiring, but we need to acknowledge that some people never reach a point where they love exercising. Often, if we keep trying different exercise options—from swimming to cycling to soccer to lifting weights to rowing to walking the dog—eventually we'll find an activity that we find enjoyable in and of itself. But sometimes that just isn't the case.

Russ loves hiking, but in itself that's not enough to keep his body as fit as he'd like. So in order to keep his upper-body muscles strong, Russ goes to the gym and lifts weights. But unlike Joe, Russ has never found this activity enjoyable. Russ likes having completed a workout at the gym—but he never actually enjoys doing it. So the point is, we can make life easier for ourselves if we find a way of exercising that's enjoyable in itself, but even if we don't enjoy the exercise, we can still do it because it's important and meaningful and life-enhancing. And we can at least enjoy the after-effects of having done it—that sense of energy and satisfaction and accomplishment, and the knowledge that we're taking care of ourselves.

We can draw three main principles from Joseph's story:

1. We spend our whole life making willingness choices.
2. Once we start saying yes, it gets easier to say yes again and again.
3. If we say yes often enough, our life starts to tip in a totally new direction.

No one can tell you whether to say yes or no. No one can tell you which goals are important to you, and no one can tell you what your particular tipping point is. But one simple rule of thumb, if you follow it, will make your life richer and more meaningful: *find a way to say yes as often as possible to the things you care about.*

Saying yes won't always be easy. If we want intimacy, we must choose to say yes to the risk of rejection. If we want success at a diet, we must choose to say yes to the risk of failure. If we want to improve our life, we must choose to say yes to something new and unpredictable, and to the inevitable feelings of anxiety that accompany change.

Jan's story: the "no diet" tipping point

Jan feels lonely. She works all day on her feet selling clothes. The customers treat her as if she is nothing more than a servant. People try on clothes and return them off their hangers and inside out, and Jan has to fix them. At the end of the day, she finds half-empty soft drink cans and milkshake cups in the shop under shelves because people can't be bothered throwing them in the bin.

Nobody thanks Jan when she does a great job of helping customers or keeping the shop tidy. So Jan finds a way to thank herself. During her breaks, she goes to her favorite coffee shop and buys a brownie or some other treat. That brownie seems magical. It lifts her right out of her gloom.

Jan's family, and especially her mother, have been pushing her to lose weight for years now. Even her best friend, Alicia, can't go more than 60 minutes without offering some diet advice. Alicia has always been thin and has no idea what Jan's life is like. Yet that doesn't stop her from parroting the latest advice from the most recent women's health magazine. This week Alicia is going on about the high-protein diet. Last week it was all about eating a lot of small snacks instead of one big meal. The week before it was all about soup. Jan wishes Alicia would just stop giving her advice. Why can't anybody accept her the way she is?

One day, like so many before, Jan decides to go on a diet. This time she manages to stay on the diet for two weeks, and even loses 5 pounds. Then, one day at work, Jan is trying to help a customer find the right dress. She's been helping the customer for about 10 minutes when the customer's phone rings. The customer interrupts Jan by answering the phone as if Jan wasn't even there, and starts talking and laughing about something. Jan waits. And waits. Finally, Jan starts to move away to help someone else, but this customer signals her to stay, despite still being on the phone. She raises a hand as if to say, "Don't go away." Jan's face flushes with anger, but what can she do? She has to stand there, waiting dumbly like a servant.

Fifty minutes later, Jan is on her break in the mall, looking at the delicious brownies in the coffee shop display case. Maybe she could go off her diet just this once. Her willingness scale is shown in Figure 6.

On the one hand, she wants to lose weight in order to please her family and friends, but that seems like an unappealing goal right now, given she already spends so much time pleasing others. On the other hand, she can eat the brownie and instantly feel better, instantly push away all the feeling of being insulted and alone.

Jan chooses the brownie.

• Feeling insulted
• Feeling lonely

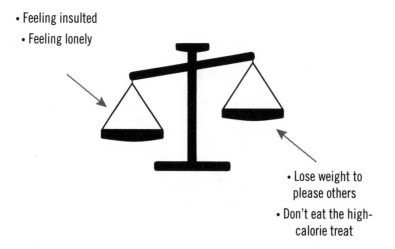

• Lose weight to please others
• Don't eat the high-calorie treat

FIGURE 6: Jan's willingness scale. Losing weight isn't worth the distress. Jan eats a brownie to comfort herself. What would you choose in this situation?

It's up to you

No one has the right to judge or criticize Jan. It's her choice and her life. Nobody has the right to tell her she should skip the treat or lose weight.

This is a central theme of this book: *you* choose your life direction, not us, not your family, not your friends. If you decide you want to lose weight, this book will help. If your goal isn't to lose weight, but rather to explore the world and make your life more enjoyable and meaningful, this book will help too. And if your goal is self-acceptance, whether you lose weight or not, then yes, this book will also help you with that. How can this be? Because this book is based on the ACT model, which is all about helping you to live a life *you* care about, supporting the goals *you* choose to create such a life.

One thing we learned in Chapter 1 is that it's important to link goals to life values. Jan's desire to lose weight is not linked to what she cares about. At present, she is only dieting because others are pressuring her. This is not really a core value. Jan is a whole, complete and complex person, with many values. She wants to develop loving, intimate relationships, have good times with her friends, learn about history and culture, and travel the world. Her current goal—losing weight to please others—doesn't link with any of these core values of love, intimacy, learning or adventure.

Jan's story 2: the "diet" tipping point

Jan has gone on for years like this, alternating between strict dieting and bingeing, but lately she's been mostly just bingeing—she's pretty much given up on dieting. But then something happens to change her life. She starts experiencing headaches that won't go away. This goes on for weeks. At first she doesn't tell anybody, but gradually she begins to fear the worst: a brain tumor. She surfs the net looking for information. Some websites say being overweight makes it more likely to get cancer. She begins to get angry with herself for having let herself go. "I made myself sick," she thinks.

She goes to see her doctor, hoping he'll reassure her. Instead, the doctor is cautious and gives her a large number of tests, including a brain scan. Waiting for these results is the longest week of her life. Finally, the results come back. Negative. The test results are negative. No tumor! The doctor believes her headaches are stress-related. "I just escaped death," she thinks.

That's when things change for Jan. She decides that caring for herself is not something to do just for other people. She wants to lose weight for herself, for her own health and wellbeing, not for anybody else. Jan's weight loss is now connected to deeply held values. That tips her willingness scale, as illustrated in Figure 7. Now she is committed to her health goals. This means that when she feels lonely or experiences an insulting customer at work, she can choose to interrupt her habitual eating of comfort food. She can choose instead to open up and make room for those difficult thoughts and feelings, and let them flow through her—neither struggling with them nor getting swept away by them. Over time, her willingness scale tips toward health.

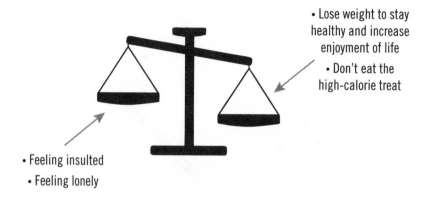

- Lose weight to stay healthy and increase enjoyment of life
- Don't eat the high-calorie treat

- Feeling insulted
- Feeling lonely

FIGURE 7: Losing weight is worth the distress. Jan passes up the brownie and allows the feelings of loneliness and not being special to flow through her— to come and stay and go in their own good time.

Embracing your distress and your goals

There's a single word that sums up these life-enhancing tipping-point decisions. It's one of the smallest and simplest words in the English language: *and*. A life-enhancing tipping point can occur when we recognize that our distress *and* our valued goals can go together. Jan was willing to make room for her feelings of loneliness *and* stick to her weight-loss goals. Joseph was willing to make room for his feelings of insecurity *and* go to the gym. The word "and" can be contrasted with a word that often seems to limit us: *but*. For example, Jan might have thought, "I'd like to stick to my weight-loss goals *but* I feel lonely." With that one word—"but"—she would have turned her feelings into the enemy of her weight-loss goals. Figure 8 on the next page shows that you can have feelings and be willing to feel them in order to move toward what you care about.

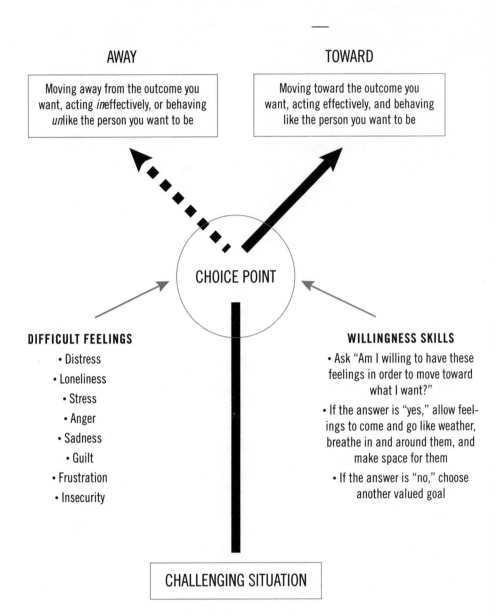

AWAY

Moving away from the outcome you want, acting *in*effectively, or behaving *un*like the person you want to be

TOWARD

Moving toward the outcome you want, acting effectively, and behaving like the person you want to be

CHOICE POINT

DIFFICULT FEELINGS

- Distress
- Loneliness
- Stress
- Anger
- Sadness
- Guilt
- Frustration
- Insecurity

WILLINGNESS SKILLS

- Ask "Am I willing to have these feelings in order to move toward what I want?"
- If the answer is "yes," allow feelings to come and go like weather, breathe in and around them, and make space for them
- If the answer is "no," choose another valued goal

CHALLENGING SITUATION

FIGURE 8: Making space for your emotions allows you to accept and move beyond them through mindful choice

EXERCISE: **FEELING DISTRESS**

In this exercise, you will see that willingness does not involve "gritting your teeth and bearing" the emotions. It is a mindful way of carrying emotions and making space for them. When we experience emotions willingly, they cease to be toxic.

We are going to ask you to experience some distress, in the service of practicing willingness. To do this, we need you to think about a fight with another person. We chose this example because research shows that we tend to engage in comfort eating after thinking about a fight. So if we practice willingness in this situation, we will be better able to manage our emotional eating after other stressful situations.

To begin, you choose the size of the willingness jump, that is, choose how emotionally confronting the memory of the fight is. Here are some examples.

- No willingness: don't think about a fight
- Less confronting: minor fight with an acquaintance
- More confronting: minor fight with a loved one
- Highly confronting: major fight with a loved one

Think about the fight now and the feelings that it brings up. Really get in touch with one core feeling related to the fight. Think about the fight and:

Allow the feeling. See if you can just allow the feeling to be there. Just make space for it, even if you don't like it.

Notice the feeling. With curiosity, notice where the feeling is in your body. Where does it start and stop? Is it moving or still?

Breathe into the feeling. Imagine your breath flowing in and around the feeling.

Physicalize the feeling. Imagine the feeling is an object. How big is it? What is its temperature? Hot, warm, cold? What color? What is its texture? Smooth? Rough?

Normalize. Say to yourself, "This is a normal feeling." Fear and desire are two sides of the same coin. When you really care about something, you are bound to be afraid of losing it or messing up somehow.

Willingness involves a mindful, accepting, open relationship to feelings. When we are willing, emotions no longer push us around. We are left with choice.

Tipping toward yes

The last two chapters have shown that trying to avoid or get rid of distress is often the cause of our problems, rather than the solution. We've also shown you a powerful alternative to emotional avoidance: *willingness*—the willingness to open up and make room for uncomfortable thoughts and feelings, to allow them to flow through you freely.

We each have to discover for ourselves what tips us toward health and wellbeing. Each person's willingness path is unique. The second half of this book will help you find that path, but before we can move to taking action, we must overcome two major barriers to willingness. The first barrier we've spoken of already: overcoming our emotional avoidance with willingness. Now we'll move on to the second major barrier: unhelpful beliefs.

In the chapters that follow, we'll show you how to break through such unhelpful beliefs, and start tipping more and more of your life toward yes.

SUMMARY: IF YOU WISH TO LOSE WEIGHT . . .

DO MORE OF THIS	DO LESS OF THIS
Recognize that you don't have to wait until you have the "right" feelings to start achieving your weight-loss goals. You can make room for distress *and* pursue your goals.	Hold on tightly to thoughts that you can't start your weight-loss goals until you have the "right" feelings, until you feel confident or motivated or in the mood.
Remember the *and:* you can feel discomfort *and* do what's important to you.	Get stuck on the *but*: hold tightly to thoughts such as "I'd like to pursue my goals, *but* it's too uncomfortable."
Find ways to tip your willingness scale to yes. Choose goals that challenge you but aren't too difficult or too far out of your comfort zone.	Hold tight to the idea that you must start with a large, highly challenging goal, and refuse to make small changes.

4.

ESCAPING THE CAGE

What if we told you that you probably underestimate your own ability to accomplish life-enhancing goals? Would you be insulted or would you feel hope? Whatever your reaction, we ask you to now consider two lines of scientific research that suggest you, and many people, probably underestimate what they are capable of doing.

The first way we know people underestimate themselves is from the phenomenon of placebos. In research, a placebo involves giving people something with no medical benefit—say, a sugar pill—and then telling them it will help in some way. The pill has no physical power to help, yet when people are given a placebo, they can still change as if they've taken something real. They experience reductions in pain and depression, and improvements in health. So clearly, if the pill has no power to help, then it's not the pill causing the improvement. Rather, the power is in the person. The people already had the potential to improve their life, they just needed a push—the placebo—to make it happen.

The second way we know people underestimate themselves is the self-fulfilling prophecy. Let's say we could convince everybody at your workplace that you're brilliant (on the off-chance they don't already believe this). What would happen next? Research suggests that if people expected you to perform well, you would in fact start to perform better. You might even perform brilliantly. In general, if teachers believe students are really smart, those students tend to perform better. If drill sergeants are told that soldiers are particularly good, those soldiers perform better. If your boss thinks you're brilliant, you'll be likely to perform better.

What the placebo and self-fulfilling prophecy studies tell us is that people always have it in them to succeed. They just don't know it. When you give them a fake pill or simply get others to believe in them, they perform better. They haven't changed, really. They just believe in themselves. They have hope.

There's a gap between what we're capable of and what we actually do. We're capable of losing weight, and of exercising regularly, yet we often don't do it. Instead we doubt ourselves and often fail to take action.

Pop psychology tells us that the way to fight difficult thoughts is to try to think positively and feel confident. Yet in Chapter 2 we showed that our attempts to control our own thoughts and feelings often fail. For example, we try to fight loneliness by comfort eating, and end up gaining weight and feeling worse about ourselves. Then we start a new diet and try to battle our self-doubt by saying something like, "No matter what happens, I won't fail this time. I can do this." But eventually the diet gets hard and the self-doubting thoughts come back: "Maybe I can't do this?," we might think. "Maybe I'll never lose weight?" Eventually, we lose the battle with our self-doubts and, at that point, may give up the diet. Does this cycle sound familiar?

As we learned in the previous chapter, the solution to dealing with difficult internal experience is not to fight, but to accept that the battle can never be won and to let go of the struggle. This chapter will show you how you can use acceptance and mindfulness skills to break the cycle between negative thoughts and self-defeating behavior.

ESCAPING THE CAGE

In the last chapter we mentioned that your mind can be one of the barriers to you trying something different. So now we're going to show you how. We'll uncover how our own mind can put us into a cage. Then we'll show you that the solution to escaping the cage isn't to bend the bars or destroy the cage. Rather, the solution is to see the bars for what they are—judgments that come and go—and then simply walk through them. Let's start this process by taking a look at John's story.

John's story: living in a cage

Around seventh grade, John became overweight. People around him started to act cruelly. They'd say, "Ew, he's ugly," and they'd call him Scarface because of his acne. The boys would tease him by acting as if he was gay and imitating him with a high-pitched voice. He was called "pig," "lardass," and almost every bad name you could think of. It got so bad he started skipping school.

John's an adult now, so you'd think he'd get over the past, but he can't. He still thinks about those days in high school. He wonders how he might have turned out differently if he hadn't been teased. He fantasizes about traveling back in time and doing something mean to those kids.

At 34, John is stuck. He just feels like he's destined to be a fat, ugly, lonely loser. Everything he wants in life seems out of reach:

- He wants to lose weight, but thinks he doesn't have enough willpower.
- He wants to feel comfortable with himself, but he hates his fat stomach.
- He wants to take better care of himself, but he thinks he doesn't have the time.
- He wants to fall in love, but he's sure that deep down there's something wrong with him. What if he meets someone and gets his hopes up and then they just crush him with rejection?
- He wants a new direction, but what if he quits the job he hates and can't get another one? Or what if the next job he gets turns out to be even worse than the one he has now?
- He wants to fix his life but he thinks it's screwed up beyond repair.

Cage builders

John feels stuck. We've all been there. To understand how to "walk through" this cage we create, we must start by understanding what causes it in the first place. Any mental cage is due to two things:

1. Society
2. The activity of our mind

CAGE BUILDER 1: SOCIETY

John was bullied by his social group. When it comes to being bullied as an adolescent, the bullying is often obvious: it's said out loud and directly to the victim. But when it comes to our weight, the bully is less obvious. The bullies are people in our community or culture who won't say things out loud, but will imply that if we're overweight, it's because there's something wrong with us, that we're weak-willed, defective or abnormal.

Indeed, the idea that being overweight is due to weakness is so pervasive that it's spawned a multibillion-dollar industry that seeks to overcome our "weaknesses" by giving us "quick and easy" diets. We're sold powders and "guilt-free shakes" that taste like toothpaste, as well as "detox" drinks that make us go to the toilet 20 times a day. We're promised ultra-low-calorie ice cream that's supposed to taste like cookies and cream but really tastes more like cold mud. And what's the basic premise underlying all this advertising? We need something "quick and easy" because we don't have the willpower to do anything else.

Our society has declared it unacceptable to insult others because of their race or religion, but in many situations it's still acceptable to insult people about their weight. This is what psychologists call a stigmatizing environment, because the messages we get from our fellow adults leave us believing we really are broken or defective.

Of course, it's crazy to think that being overweight indicates something is wrong with us. More than half the population is overweight, so being overweight is actually *normal* in our environment. There are plenty of good environmental reasons for this, including easy access to high-calorie foods and culture-wide decreases in physical activity. For example, we don't have to chase a gazelle for 10 miles before finally catching it, killing it and eating it—we can drive through McDonald's for our food.

Yet knowing this doesn't really help us, does it? We still believe we need to look like anorexic runway models or beefy bodybuilders to be okay. Next time you're in a crowded place—say, a supermarket—cast your eye around to see how real people with real bodies look. Almost nobody comes close to the ideal. We're humans, not caricatures of Barbie or Ken.

Unfortunately, we believe all too readily that if we're not at the "right" weight, it means we're weak-willed or flawed or unlikable or unlovable or defective or inferior or inadequate. And that's when we start to get into real trouble. We come to believe that the only way we can become lovable or adequate or worthwhile is to lose weight. And this in turn leads to desperate ongoing attempts to lose weight with fad diets. But here's what usually happens when we try:

1. We rarely if ever lose as much weight as we want.
2. Even if we *do* lose the weight, we struggle to *keep* it off—and as soon as it goes back on, we immediately beat ourselves up again.
3. Even if we *do* manage to lose all the weight we want, and keep it off, our self-critical mind is rarely satisfied for long; it soon finds plenty of other ways to judge us as unlovable, unworthy or inadequate.

How can we learn to achieve our weight-loss goals through self-kindness and acceptance when our society tells us to be self-loathing and critical? We'd love to change society. We hope this book will *begin* to change society. But we're alive now and can't wait for society to change. We need to break free from society's cage now. And we can; society can only cage us with the help of our own minds.

CAGE BUILDER 2: OUR MIND

We can think of the mind as a super-duper problem-solving machine, constantly spotting problems and figuring out how to solve them. The mind isn't there to make you feel good, it's there to detect threats. It has developed to help us survive.

The mind solves problems of safety. "Is this place safe?" it asks, or "What's that blob in the distance? Is it a lion?" or "Is this fruit safe to eat?" Importantly, in our violent historical past, a major threat to our safety was other people. Thus our mind is especially prepared to see other people as dangerous problems to be solved: "Is that person going to hurt me? What's his intention? Good or bad?" The mind also solves problems of food, water and shelter: "How do I get food? Which foods will help me survive?" (In other words, which foods are high in calories?) It also solves the problems of finding a mate: "Is this person reliable? Trustworthy? Strong?"

The mind is especially sensitive to problems of status, because having high status means you'll probably have more resources (better food, more money, more power, better social alliances) and thus a better chance of survival. So the mind is always asking questions like, "Is this person better than me? Does that man have a higher status than this man? Am I thinner than her?"

Three principles can help us understand our problem-solving minds:

1. OUR MINDS ARE ESSENTIAL TO US

The mind is a machine that detects danger. We need it to tell us when there's a problem or threat. We'd be unable to survive without it.

2. OUR MINDS CAN'T BE TURNED OFF

If you could turn your mind-machine off, you wouldn't live very long. Imagine if you had a switch on the back of your head and you could flip it down to turn off your mind. One day you might be feeling particularly relaxed and safe, so you flip the switch. You feel great. You're totally peaceful and free from anxiety.

But what happens if a genuine danger shows up? Perhaps a snake slithers into your garden, or you have to cross a busy highway, or a mugger is approaching you. Would you know to protect yourself? No, because your mind wouldn't be evaluating the environment for danger.

3. OUR MINDS ARE OFTEN NEGATIVE

Think about it. If your mind is the danger alarm that keeps you alive, would you rather have it go off too often or too rarely? If it goes off too much, you'll often be running from your own shadow and from things that aren't real threats. That's bad, but it isn't as bad as the alternative: if it were to go off too infrequently and fail to go off when there was a danger, then you might be killed. You only get to make that mistake once.

The mind has evolved to help us survive. But what if there's a flaw with it? What if it actually hinders us too—particularly in the context of our weight-loss goals? Let's now look at this possibility, and make sense of how our mind may be getting in our way. The fact is, the problem-solving mind is great when it's focused on the outside world and on survival. Unfortunately, though, the mind is restless. It starts to turn inwards, onto ourselves. This is the problem. Just like it judges the world as good and bad, it starts to judge our body as good or bad, and our personality as a problem to be solved.

The mind sets its keen focus on body parts like our thighs and stomach, and then asks, "Are they too flabby?" Your mind can see every part of your body as problematic: "Your nose, your ears, your lips. Are these ugly?" The mind takes no prisoners and leaves no part of your body unexamined.

Here's an example from our author Ann's experience, where self-judgments rapidly changed her relationship with her body from positive to negative.

Ann's story: Sally and the pot belly

I don't know about you, but my mind betrays me pretty regularly when it comes to my body. Let me tell you a story about the last time this happened. It was fairly recently, around my 40th birthday. This is a milestone age for most women, when they ask themselves about the meaning of life and other profound matters. My existential crisis was focused on only one thing: my pot belly. Making its appearance in my thirties, it gained significance 60 pounds and two pregnancies later. No longer was I young or beautiful or particularly desirable, I thought. But my denial of the aging process was strong. And so, despite the evidence staring me down, I was determined to turn back time.

I made a commitment to myself: over the next year I'd do whatever it took to get the body I'd always wanted. Maybe then I wouldn't have to be 40. Or look 40. Or feel 40. I was inspired. I began searching through magazines to find the perfect body, and, to my delight, it wasn't long before I found the leanest, perfectly proportioned cover girl alive. So up she went on the fridge, in all her glory. I (stupidly) showed all my friends the picture and informed them confidently that in a year I planned to look just like her. I felt excited and motivated.

And so, the very next day, after my 40th birthday party (where I put away a large amount of chocolate birthday cake as a last hurrah), the work began. I disciplined myself to five hard workouts a week and a low-carb, high-protein diet. It was hell, but I was determined.

The torture had been going on for about three months when finally it happened: I looked in the mirror and thought, "Wow . . . it's really working! I'm finally starting to look okay. My belly is flattening out." It felt amazing. I could now officially tell myself that even if I *was* 40, I didn't have to believe it.

Until the day I paid a visit to my ironing lady, Sally. It was as I handed my basket to her that it happened. Sally poked my belly with her finger, and said, "Oh Ann, love, are you expecting another one?"

I put my head down, laughed it off and scurried back to the car only to consume myself with embarrassment and loathing about my disgusting pig-like belly that only hours before I had so proudly showed off. There was no more denial. In that moment, I never felt so fat, pathetic and old. Maybe it really was time to give up.

MIND OVER MATTER

Our mind can radically change how we think about our body, even if our body doesn't radically change. Our mind turns our body into a problem to be solved. If our mind has decided we're too fat, then naturally the solution seems to be to diet. There's now a multibillion-dollar diet and exercise industry that seeks to fix the "fat problem" your mind has identified. This industry feeds the mind what it wants to hear. The "flat-stomach diet plan" is great if your mind has decided your stomach is the problem. The "quick and easy diet plan" is great if your mind has concluded you don't have enough motivation. The "revolutionary new diet plan" is great if your mind has concluded all past diet plans are the problem and you just need something new.

We bounce from diet to diet, hoping that eventually we'll find the solution to the problems our mind keeps generating, hoping we can fix all the parts in ourselves that our mind has judged not good enough.

Sarah's story: the perfect girl

By our current society's standards, Sarah is perfect. A beautiful 22-year-old, she's neither too fat nor too thin. She dresses well and always appears stylish. Her makeup is well applied, her hair always done perfectly and her nails polished. And Sarah is a nice girl too—always pleasant toward others. You'd never hear her complain or say something bad about anyone. To top it all off, Sarah is a high achiever: at school she won swimming races, got great grades and edited the school newspaper. People look at Sarah and think, "Wow, she's got it all."

Yet Sarah doesn't think so. She often feels there is something not quite right with her and berates herself for things she's said or done. Sarah feels like she's always falling short—never being supportive enough to her friends, never working as hard as she can, never looking quite right. When it comes to her body, Sarah is particularly harsh—if only she could get a bit more shape in her arms, or maybe a few more pounds off . . . It's never enough. Sarah keeps herself on a tight leash and only allows herself certain portion sizes and calorie-controlled meals.

At times, Sarah can't take it any more, and she'll find herself in the middle of a binge—multiple slices of toast, cheese, ice cream and anything else she can find in the fridge. When Sarah binges she feels alive and free, like she's giving the finger to the world and finally having something *she* wants. Until her mind starts beating her up, telling her she should be more self-disciplined, telling her she is broken.

Your mind: the unreliable adviser

You can think of your mind as an unreliable adviser. Sometimes it tells you useful things, sometimes what it says is not so useful. For example, it may offer you the advice that you're too fat, too lazy and too undisciplined. Maybe it will advise you that you'll never succeed. It can be quite convincing.

Can you think of someone who once gave you bad advice? Maybe they were totally convinced they were right, but they turned out to be completely wrong. Perhaps they didn't have your best interests at heart, or they didn't fully understand your life situation. Either way, take a moment to consider how someone can be absolutely certain about what you should do in a certain situation, and yet that person can be totally wrong.

The human mind is like that. It can be absolutely convincing, 100 percent certain that it knows best—and yet turn out to be completely wrong. Imagine your mind is an adviser that follows you around all day. That by itself would be very annoying. But imagine it was even worse. Imagine this adviser would, at unexpected times, put a sign in front of your face with some short piece of advice for you. The sign would be so close to your face that you could see nothing but what the sign told you. Here are a few examples of signs from a mind having a bad day.

YOU ARE NOT GOOD ENOUGH

DON'T SCREW UP

YOU LOOK FAT

WHAT'S WRONG WITH YOU?

Think how hard it would be to walk around with these signs always in your face. You wouldn't be able to see anything but the signs. You'd miss important information in the world around you. You might turn down a wrong street or walk into traffic. You might fail to notice a friend and say hello. You might not be able to enjoy your lunch or respond to someone who needs your help.

We can't get rid of this adviser, of course—it's part of our biology. We can't stop it from showing us the signs. But what we can do is learn to see the signs from a certain wise distance. Imagine if you could step back from the signs, so that they are no longer in your face blocking your view. You could still read the signs and you wouldn't always like what they said, but at least they wouldn't be overpowering. If you had this wise distance, you'd have more freedom to look around you and decide how you want to act. The signs wouldn't dominate your view so much.

Fusion

When our thoughts dominate our awareness, or our actions, or both, we call it *fusion*. When things are fused together, they're connected to each other very powerfully. So, if we're fused with our thoughts, it means they're having a major impact on us. It may be that they dominate our awareness—such as when we are worrying, or stressing out, or dwelling on the past, or simply "lost in thought." Or it may be they dominate our actions—such as when our mind tells us to eat that cream doughnut or skip that exercise.

So fusion with our thoughts isn't always helpful. Imagine we saw the world through a pair of shit-colored goggles: everything would look like shit. Something similar happens when we fuse with highly judgmental thoughts. Suppose we look at our bodies while fused with thoughts such as "Ugh! I look awful! I hate this body!" Then our body seems truly awful; we forget all the wonderful aspects of it—like the way it helps us to see, hear, touch, taste, smell, breathe, walk and talk. This kind of fusion happens all the time to all of us. We may fuse with judgments that our job sucks, or our boss is an asshole, or our father-in-law is crazy, or our children are ungrateful, or our president is an idiot. And each time we do so, we are effectively looking at the world through those shit-colored goggles. This is perfectly normal and natural; we all do it, repeatedly; but it doesn't help us. In fact, fusion dramatically hinders us and stands as a barrier to our weight-loss and other goals.

So our job is to become aware of this stealthy barrier called fusion, begin to notice when it's paying us a visit, and then learn skills to overcome it so that our thoughts no longer stand in our way. We'll learn how to step back from our thoughts and look at them, rather than through them. This will allow us to have difficult thoughts while at the same time moving toward values.

FUSION VERSUS DEFUSION

Fusion means our awareness and our actions are dominated by our thoughts.

Defusion means we break the dominance of our thoughts, we see their true nature; we realize they are nothing more nor less than words and pictures in our head.

Recognize your "I'm not good enough" story

The "I'm not good enough" story is the best-kept secret on the planet. We're all walking around with multiple versions of it—*I'm fat, I'm stupid, I'm incompetent, I can't cope, I'm not smart enough, I'm nothing special, I don't fit in, I'm boring, I'm unlikable, I'm unlovable, I keep screwing up, I haven't achieved enough, I'm too lazy, I'm selfish, I'm a pushover, I'm a control freak, I'm too judgmental, I'm a bad mother/father/son/daughter, I'm not attractive, I'm too egotistical, I'm too anxious, I'm too depressed, I eat too much, I don't exercise enough, I never get it right, It's all my fault, I've got no motivation/discipline/willpower*, and so on.

Even though we all have multiple versions of this tale, almost no one ever owns up to having such thoughts. At least not very often. And why not? Because we live in a culture obsessed with positive thinking, a society that teaches us to see negative thoughts as unnatural and harmful. And if we do own up to such thoughts, there's a good chance someone will tag us as mentally unwell and tell us we're suffering from depression, anxiety or low self-esteem.

So naturally folks are reluctant to own up to thinking this way. But if you get to know someone well and look beneath the surface, then chances are you'll find that even the most apparently positive, happy, confident people have no shortage of "I'm not good enough" stories going through their head. Indeed, while traveling round the world giving hundreds of ACT workshops to public and professionals alike, we have now asked well over 25,000 people, "Is there anyone in this room who doesn't have at least one version of the 'I'm not good enough' story that shows up at times and pushes you around, brings you down, or holds you back?" So far, no one has ever said yes.

Of course, "I'm not good enough" stories take different forms. Sometimes they're long rambling monologues about all the ways we don't measure up, while at other times they just pop up as one-word thoughts, such as "Idiot!" And while at times we can be very aware of these stories, often we're so used to them we don't even realize our minds are talking to us this way.

EXERCISE: DEFUSING FROM THE STORY

To help you learn defusion, we need to first experience the opposite: fusion. So, we'd like you now to pick an unhelpful thought and get really fused with it. We want you to totally buy into it and believe it. This will probably make you feel bad initially, but we hope you're willing to feel uncomfortable for a few moments in order to learn something useful. Once you've fused with the thought, we'll show you how to *defuse* from it.

We suggest you pick some version of the "I'm not good enough" story to work with. So pick a thought from one of your most potent versions of the "I'm not good enough" story and put it into a short sentence, for example, "I'm too fat" or "I'm not smart enough." Now see if you can *fuse* with it. In other words, for the next 10 seconds, see if you can totally buy into this thought—believe it as much as you possibly can.

Now it's time to try to create some defusion. First, silently repeat the same thought to yourself, but with this phrase in front of it: "I'm having the thought that..." For example, "I'm having the thought that I'm fat."

Notice what happens.

Now do that once again, but this time use a slightly longer phrase: "I notice I'm having the thought that..." For example, "I notice I'm having the thought that I'm fat."

Notice what happens.

As you tried those exercises, did you notice yourself developing some sort of distance or detachment from the thought? A sense of separating or moving away from it, much as your hand can move away from your face? If so, you've achieved defusion. If not, try the exercise again with a different thought until you do.

Letting go of the truth game

At this point in learning to create defusion, many people protest. They say something like, "But it's true. I really am fat/stupid/selfish/lazy/unworthy/a bad mother!"

Once you hear yourself say "but it's true," you'll know you're hearing your judgmental mind. Your mind loves to solve problems and figure out what's "true" or "false." We're so proud of our minds and their incredible power that we lose sight of one simple thing: our minds are great for solving problems in the outside world, such as how to survive, but they're not so great at solving problems inside us. Our mind can spend years trying to figure out how we're flawed and how we can be "fixed," and not get anywhere.

The good news is this: we don't have to wait until our mind figures everything out before we act. Our mind is only an adviser. That's all. We don't have to let it tell us what to do. We can decide to stop listening to its judgments of true and false. Instead, we can focus on whether or not a thought is *helpful*. When difficult thoughts pop into your head, if you hold onto them tightly, get all caught up in them, allow them to push you around and dictate what you do, does that help you to behave like the person you want to be, do the things you want to do, create the life you want to live? If the answer is yes, then by all means hold onto them. But if it's no, wouldn't you like to defuse from them, regardless of whether they're true or not?

The key to defusion is simply to see the true nature of your thoughts, to see them for what they really are—neither more nor less than words and pictures. When we see that this is the basic essence of a thought—a word or picture in our head—we can let go of all those magical ideas about thoughts being harmful to us, which in turn frees us from having to fight or struggle with them.

Defusion: practice does not make perfect, but does lead to improvement

We're now going to do an exercise to help you recognize the true nature of your thoughts, to "see" them as words. (Note: although we're focusing on words here, if your thoughts more often take the form of pictures and images, you can easily modify most of these techniques to suit.)

Once you've been through the whole exercise, we'll show you a simpler method for creating defusion, but we're starting with these because they're a good training ground. They're like using floaties as you learn to swim; once you know how to do it, you can throw the floaties away.

Please give each step of the exercise a go. You may or may not be able to do what we ask of you, but just try it, and if you find you can't do it, simply acknowledge that and move on to the next one.

And please bring an attitude of curiosity and openness to these experiments. Some of the steps might not create defusion at all. Some might give you a teeny-weeny bit of defusion. Some might give you a lot of defusion. And some might actually create *fusion*! (We don't expect fusion to happen with these exercises, but sometimes it does. If it does with you, that's not a problem at all. Just acknowledge it—say to yourself, "Oh, I just *fused* with that thought!" and then move on to the next step. The great thing is, when we acknowledge to ourselves that we're fused with a thought, that in itself generally creates some defusion—it helps us step back from the thought at least a little!)

EXERCISE: PLAY WITH YOUR THOUGHTS TO DEFUSE

Let's start. This defusion exercise helps you see your thoughts as just words— nothing more, nothing less. We'd like you to begin by bringing to mind a negative self-judgment and putting it in a short sentence, such as "I am unlovable" or "I'm not thin enough."

Now imagine it as simple black text, in lower case, on a computer screen:

I am unlovable

(If you have access to one, this exercise is even more powerful if you do it for real on the computer, instead of just imagining it.) Now play around with the formatting. Space the words far apart, so there are huge gaps between them:

I   am   unlovable

Now run all the words together, so there's no space between them:

Iamunlovable

Now run the words vertically down the screen:

I

am

unlovable

Now put the words into several different fonts (and better still, if you can, in a range of different colors):

I am unlovable

I am unlovable

I am unlovable

I AM UNLOVABLE

I am unlovable

Now see if you can animate the words, the way they do in those cartoons on *Sesame Street*: imagine the words jumping up and down the screen, spinning in circles, stretching, bouncing, and so on.

Now imagine those words written in bright colorful graphics, on the cover of a children's book.

Now imagine those words created in chocolate icing on the top of a birthday cake.

Now imagine those words printed as an item on a restaurant menu.

Now imagine those words painted on a banner, trailing behind an airplane high up in the sky.

Now imagine those words scribbled in a six-year-old's handwriting on a drawing stuck to the fridge.

Now imagine those words as a tattoo on the arm of a beautiful actress or actor, like Angelina Jolie or Brad Pitt.

Now imagine those words sculpted out of rock in the garden of a modern art museum.

Now draw a stick man on a piece of paper, with a thought bubble coming out of his head, and write those words inside it. (If you can't physically do this right now, just imagine it—but at your first opportunity, please actually do it for real.)

There are many other ways to play with thoughts. The above example is visual, but you can also play with the sound. For example, you can imagine your difficult thoughts in a funny song. Imagine singing this to the tune of "Happy Birthday": "I'm so unlovable today. I'm so unlovable today. I'm so unlovable, dear Ann Bailey. I'm so unlovable today." You might also say your unhelpful thoughts using a funny voice. The point of these exercises is not to challenge the truth of the thoughts, but to see the true nature of them: to see that they are nothing more or less than words. Sometimes these words can be useful and sometimes not.

ANALYZING YOUR RESPONSE

Did you notice how the words changed as you did this exercise? Did some of their power disappear? Did you perhaps see them as just words? If so, congratulations. You've defused from the thought. In future, you'll of course fuse with it again. This is inevitable: fusion is the default setting for all humans. But you can get better and better at unhooking yourself from these thoughts, at recognizing you're fused and then promptly defusing again.

Defusion is an essential skill to develop. We urge you to practice it as much as possible. Practice playing around with the ideas above, any time, anywhere. When you realize you've been hooked by a self-limiting belief or a nasty self-judgment or a worrying thought about the future or a painful thought about the past, take a moment to defuse from it. Believe us when we say the work will be worth it. If you can master the skill of defusion you'll have developed much greater power to achieve your weight-loss goals. For reference, here's an illustration of the defusion skills we have outlined in this chapter.

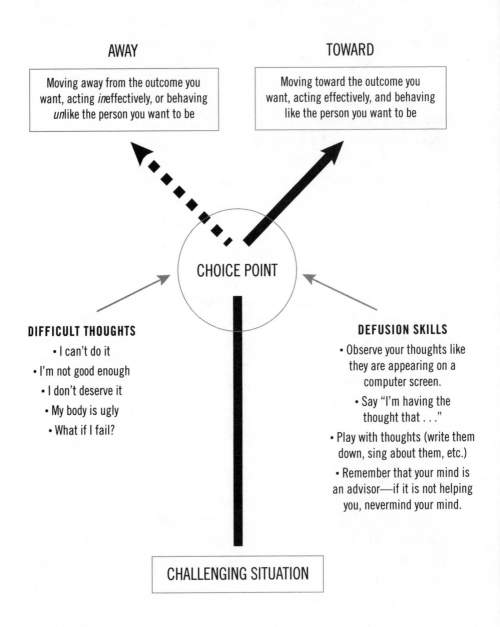

FIGURE 9: Defusion skills summary

SUMMARY: IF YOU WISH TO LOSE WEIGHT . . .

DO MORE OF THIS	DO LESS OF THIS
Recognize that all humans have a self-critical mind or what we've called a problem-solving machine. This machine beats us up sometimes. It's part of human biology.	Believe that your self-criticism is a sign there really is something wrong with you. Fail to recognize that all humans have this self-criticism machine.
Notice your "I'm not good enough" story. Give it a name.	Believe your "I'm not good enough" story. Let it dictate what you do.
Create wise distance from self-defeating thoughts by writing them down, doing something playful with them (singing them in funny voices or imagining them changing on a computer screen).	Treat whatever your mind says as the absolute truth and do whatever it says.
Practice having difficult thoughts and still doing what you care about. For example, practice exercising even when you have the thought "I'm too lazy to exercise."	Every time a difficult thought comes up, stop doing what you care about.

5.
HARNESSING THE POWER OF FLEXIBILITY

Nothing is softer or more flexible than water, yet nothing can resist it.

—Lao Tzu

Elise's story: declaring war on weight

Elise is ready to start her diet on Monday. She swears to herself she won't fail like last time. She'll follow the diet exactly and eat nothing that's forbidden. She feels determined and focused, like a boxer just before a major fight.

The diet requires her to eliminate most carbohydrates: no pasta, no bread and definitely no pastries. She loves pasta but she's ready to make the sacrifice. On Sunday night, against her husband's strong protests, she cleans out the cupboards and throws away all the carb-rich foods.

On Monday morning, she wakes excited to start the first day of her new regime. She makes the shake that she'll substitute for her breakfast. It tastes a bit grainy and artificial, but she reckons she can drink it. She'll do anything to shed 20 pounds.

Then she remembers she's supposed to have lunch with a friend on Tuesday. There's no way she can go to their favorite Indian restaurant on this diet. There are no other good restaurants nearby. She'll have to cancel.

RIGID DIET RULES

Elise is determined and will probably lose weight, but do you think she'll be able to sustain the weight loss? We would guess not, because it's clear that Elise is under the control of strong and rigid diet rules. A rigid rule has an all or nothing quality to it and is generally accompanied by words like "should," "have to," "must," "ought," "right," "wrong," "good," "bad," "mustn't" and "can't." It's a bit like walking around with your own personal dictator inside your head laying down the rules, running your life, warning you that terrible things will happen if you dare defy their orders. We all sometimes cling to rigid diet rules in order to avoid losing control. But do such rules actually work the way we hope they will?

The research suggests not. People who follow rigid diet rules are actually more likely to binge-eat and have a higher weight. In other words, rigid diet rules not only fail to protect us from weight gain, they may actually increase our weight.

Rigid diet rules fail because they make us insensitive to what we want and need. For example, rigid dieters will eat diet foods even when those foods don't taste good. They'll ignore the feedback from their bodies and eat a diet that makes them feel tired and run down. The diet rules lead them to forgo pleasures, such as an enjoyable meal with friends. Typically, while on the diet, they feel a tremendous burden, a sense that something is lacking, or a feeling of missing out—which often leads them to resent those very dietary rules they've imposed on themselves.

The following one-minute quiz will help you to identify if you sometimes hold on tightly to rigid diet rules.

ONE-MINUTE QUIZ: **DO YOU HAVE FUSED DIET RULES?**

Recall how in Chapter 4 we defined fusion as being dominated by some sort of thought: an idea, a belief, an assumption, a prediction, a judgment, a rule. When we fuse with a rule, it has a huge impact on our behavior—we either believe it's absolutely true or we feel like we *have to* obey it, or both. And typically, if we don't follow the rule with which we've fused, we feel bad about ourselves (because we fuse with harsh self-criticism).

Now we invite you to explore the diet rules you sometimes fuse with (that is, you believe them, or hold on tightly to them, or worry about them, or allow them to push you around and dictate what you do).

DIET RULE	HOW OFTEN DO YOU AGREE WITH THE DIET RULE?				
	NEVER	RARELY	SOMETIMES	OFTEN	ALWAYS
Gaining even a small amount of weight is a sign I'm failing at my diet.	0	1	2	3	4
I need guilt to motivate me to lose weight.	0	1	2	3	4
I need to eat diet foods even when I don't like how they taste.	0	1	2	3	4
I must skip meals to lose weight.	0	1	2	3	4
I must be on a diet plan to lose weight.	0	1	2	3	4
Dieting means forbidding myself from eating certain foods (e.g., dessert, carbs).	0	1	2	3	4
A diet plan needs to offer me quick success.	0	1	2	3	4
Dieting requires me to deprive myself.	0	1	2	3	4

Did you answer 2 or above for many of these questions? If so, then you might be somebody who fuses with rigid diet rules. Which of the rules did you rate the highest? That is the one to keep an eye on. It is the rule that is most likely to push you around if you let it.

Elise's story 2: a lifetime of rigid diet rules

Elise clings to rigid diet rules because she secretly fears she's low in willpower, that she lacks self-discipline, that she could lose control at any time. And once she loses control, she fears, she'll fall apart. It seems to her that her only protection is to cling tightly to those rigid diet rules. These simple strings of words offer so much hope and reassurance to Elise:

- Skip breakfast
- No snacking
- No dessert
- No pasta

And for a short time, these four "commandments" really do work! To her great sense of relief, Elise genuinely manages to avoid the "bad" foods she craves. However, as the days pass, she starts to feel increasingly irritable and hungry. But the commandment says "Thou must skip breakfast!" so she goes without and has a coffee instead. Sometimes Elise just feels like treating herself to a small dessert, but the commandment says "Thou shalt not eat dessert." She listens carefully to these words, at the beginning, for like an ancient prophet, her mind promises her good things will come if she follows the commandments dutifully. But it's exhausting. Especially as new words start showing up for her:

- I'll just eat this one pasta meal and then tomorrow I'll be very strict again.
- I don't have time to go to the gym today. I'll go tomorrow.
- I can't help myself. I have no motivation.

The other side of diet rules: reasons

Elise is doing what so many of us do. When the rigid diet rules fail, as they so often do, we switch to a new verbal activity called *creating reasons for failing*. We're all taught from an extremely young age to come up with reasons for everything we do. If, as a child, you were asked, "Why did you hit Sally?" and you said, "I don't know," the adult would keep asking you why until you came up with a good reason. We're encouraged to come up with reasons for everything, and it's only natural that we therefore come up with reasons for *not* doing things. Use the one-minute quiz below to help you identify the reasons you favor when it comes to both breaking your diet and avoiding exercise.

ONE-MINUTE QUIZ: **DO YOU GIVE REASONS FOR NOT DIETING OR EXERCISING?**

Do you make excuses for not reaching for your health goals? Do any of these sound familiar to you?

REASON FOR NOT DIETING OR EXERCISING	HOW OFTEN DO YOU BELIEVE THIS REASON FOR NOT DIETING OR EXERCISING?				
	NEVER	RARELY	SOMETIMES	OFTEN	ALWAYS
I don't have time to shop for and/or prepare a healthy meal.	0	1	2	3	4
Places to exercise are all too far away.	0	1	2	3	4
Healthy food costs too much.	0	1	2	3	4
There are few healthy options when I eat out.	0	1	2	3	4
It costs too much to exercise.	0	1	2	3	4
I don't know how to cook well enough.	0	1	2	3	4
I do not have enough willpower.	0	1	2	3	4
I don't know enough about healthy eating.	0	1	2	3	4
I don't feel motivated to exercise.	0	1	2	3	4
My family doesn't encourage me to eat healthily.	0	1	2	3	4
I'm too embarrassed to exercise.	0	1	2	3	4
Healthy foods don't taste good.	0	1	2	3	4
I don't have access to healthy food options at home or work.	0	1	2	3	4
I don't have time to exercise.	0	1	2	3	4
I've gone off my diet today, so I might as well give up for now and indulge myself.	0	1	2	3	4
I'm starting my diet tomorrow, so I'll eat as much as I want today.	0	1	2	3	4
I exercised this morning so I can eat more now.	0	1	2	3	4

Did you score 2 or higher on many of the questions? If so, you might tend to fuse with reasoning for not engaging in healthy behavior. We all generate reasons; this is one of our favorite activities as humans. The key is to notice which of these reasons is so believable that you would let it dictate what you do.

BREAKING THE RULE–REASON CYCLE

Diet rules and reason-giving don't have to control your life. Believe it or not, research has shown that you can successfully lose weight without holding on to any rules or reasons. The first step in freeing ourselves from the power of these rules and reasons is to increase our awareness of them. When we're unaware of our own self-defeating thought patterns, they exert a massive influence over our behavior, but as we increase our awareness of them, they start to lose their power over us. The two quizzes in this chapter will have helped you take the first step and made you more aware of your mind's habitual patterns of rule-making and reason-giving. Now it's time to take the next step: *observing or defusing from thoughts*.

When we truly observe our thoughts with an attitude of openness and curiosity, we see that they're nothing more or less than words and pictures. We break the cycle of diet rules and excuses. When it comes to observing or defusing our thoughts, there are basically two elements: *noticing* and *naming*.

Noticing and naming your thoughts

Noticing is something you've already practiced while reading this book. Each time you followed our instructions to pause and check out what your mind was saying, that was an instance of noticing. *Naming* simply means using words to describe whatever we've noticed. So, for example, suppose you're all caught up in a rule–reason cycle about why you can't exercise today that looks something like: *I can't do this. It's too hard.* The first step is to notice it and the second step is to name it. In other words, as soon as you're aware of the thought, you label it with words. So you might say, "Oh . . . here comes a reason" or "There's that 'too hard' story again" or, more simply, "Reason-giving."

Let's take a few moments to do some noticing and naming now. Notice and name what is showing up for you now by completing the sentences:

- Right now, I am having the thought that . . .
- Right now, I am having the feeling of . . .
- Right now, I am having the sensations . . .

Here is an example from Joseph. "Right now I'm having the thought that I want a high-calorie nut bar and I don't have time to prepare anything else. Right now I'm feeling stress and time pressure. Right now I have the sensation of tension in my stomach."

This simple noticing and naming process is enough to give Joseph a "mindful pause." It helps him to defuse from his thoughts, and in that pause, he gains the power of choice.

Noticing and naming is powerful. It can be a skill you have in your arsenal at all times that most other people will never obtain or understand. But, like anything powerful and important, this skill takes practice. It's not hard practice, but it's tricky, because during the stresses of everyday life, we forget about it. We get so caught up in all our concerns and worries that we lose touch with what we're thinking and feeling, and with what we're telling ourselves.

It's not possible to notice and name all the time, but you can focus your practice on key points in the day, and the more often you do it, the more powerful the skill becomes. For example, you could practice noticing and naming just before you make key healthy lifestyle decisions. Will you eat a high-calorie snack? Will you go to the gym? Should you get takeaway food? When you're faced with eating choices, you can rapidly check in with yourself like this:

1. NOTICE AND NAME YOUR FEELINGS
Just before you make your decision, ask yourself: "What am I feeling right now?"

2. NOTICE WHAT YOUR MIND WANTS YOU TO DO
Is it providing you with excuses for choosing an unhealthy option? Does it say "you deserve it" or "you can't help yourself"? Is it giving you a "license to eat badly"? For example, maybe it "gives you permission" to make an unhealthy choice because you exercised earlier or because you plan to starve yourself in the next few days. Watch out for your clever mind and its ability to give you reasons for doing a value-inconsistent, "away" move.

3. NAME YOUR INTENTION

Ask yourself, "What do I want to do in this situation? How do I want to treat my body?" You might say, "I want to enjoy a small amount of a treat, mindfully." Or "Right now, I want to choose the healthy option."

Noticing and naming helps you to have *flexibility* of choice: the diet rules and excuses won't be ruling you. Flexibility means you're able to persist in your health goals or change them as the situation demands. The flexible dieter doesn't ignore their body's needs. Nor do they persist with a diet that isn't working or is making them tired and miserable. We'll have much more to say about dieting flexibly below.

EXERCISE: UNDERMINING REASON-GIVING WITH THE GOAL/EXCUSES CARD

We know that practice is the way to increase our power when it comes to defusion. This simple exercise will help you in that practice, and help you move closer to your weight-loss goals. All it requires is a small index card or piece of paper that you can carry in your pocket, wallet or purse.

Doing this will help you practice the skill of defusing from your excuses in order to help you achieve your goals. When excuses no longer dominate you, you'll have more freedom of action. You, rather than that dictator in your head, will get to choose what happens next.

First pick a realistic health goal from the table below, which is divided into four general domains:

1. Improving diet
2. Increasing exercise
3. Reducing sedentary behavior—even if you exercise for 30 minutes a day, there's a chance you're quite inactive the rest of the time
4. Creating a health-enhancing environment

IMPROVING DIET	INCREASING EXERCISE	REDUCING SEDENTARY BEHAVIOR	CREATING A HEALTH-ENHANCING ENVIRONMENT
Increase awareness of what you eat by completing a food diary (see appendix)	Increase awareness of your exercise patterns by completing an exercise journal	Do things standing up rather than sitting down (e.g., reading the newspaper)	Get at least eight hours of sleep a night
Eat breakfast	Take up dancing or some other fun physical activity	Wear a pedometer and set a goal of 8,000 to 10,000 steps per day	Follow the half-plate rule (fill one half of your plate with fruit and vegetables, the other with meat and/or carbohydrates)
Reduce your salt intake	Take a regular brisk walk	Get off the couch and walk around the house during TV ad breaks	Use small containers to store your food
Shift from eating fried fast food to fresh fast food	Do regular weight training	Have standing or walking meetings at work	Put everything you plan to eat on your plate before you start eating
Get a complete physical check-up from your doctor and seek advice from a qualified dietician	Take up a team sport	Get off the bus or train early and walk the rest of the way	Use smaller plates and bowls
Eat a meal mindfully (see page 141)	Take up jogging, cycling, running, swimming or some other aerobic activity you enjoy	Walk to the shops or to work	Eat more fruit, vegetables and legumes and increase their variety
Be assertive in refusing food you're offered but don't really want	Commit to the gym on certain days of the week	Walk the children to school	Reduce distractions when eating
Eat smaller portion sizes at a restaurant (e.g., order an appetizer size rather than an entrée)	Exercise for a set amount of time (e.g., at least 175 minutes a week or 30–60 minutes on most days)	Stand up during phone calls	Watch for social influence (see page 72)
Replace a low-fiber, high-sugar breakfast cereal with a high-fiber, low-sugar one	Gradually increase your exercise time until you reach a new goal	Stand and take a break from the computer every 30 minutes	Eat mindfully with other people
Eat low-GI foods (see appendix)	Seek advice from a qualified personal trainer	Walk to your errands, or walk between them	Reduce access to unhealthy foods (don't have junk food within easy reach)
Start the meal with a food low in energy density (e.g., soup or a salad)	Train for an event (e.g., a race or competition)	Park the car further away from your destination and walk the rest of the way	Increase access to healthy foods (put a bowl of fruit on the table)
Replace foods of high energy density with foods of low energy density (see appendix)	Exercise with a friend	Use the stairs rather than the lift or escalator	Identify what time of day you feel desperately hungry and plan for this with healthy snacks
Eat more whole foods	Get out into the garden regularly or mow the lawn once a week	Stand up at work, if possible or if you don't already	Seek support from others for your health goals

You can generate a goal of your own if you prefer, but the key is to choose something you haven't been doing and you'd like to do more of. This might include exercising briefly, replacing an unhealthy breakfast with a healthier one, or drinking sparkling water instead of a sugary soft drink.

Once you've chosen your goal, write it down on your small index card or piece of paper. Make the goal specific. Describe when and where you'll do it. Then, on the other side the card, write down the excuses your mind might use to talk you out of your goal. For example, if you decide you want to go for a 20-minute walk before dinner, you might anticipate thinking, "Oh, I don't have time today." See the example goal/excuse card below. If you decide to have more vegetables with your dinner, you might watch out for excuses like "Vegetables aren't going to satisfy me" or "Vegetables are so boring." If you decide to do some vigorous exercise, you might have excuses like "I don't feel motivated today" or "I hate going to the gym."

Side 1 of card: goal	Side 2 of card: excuses
20-minute walk before dinner	I won't have time
	I'm too tired

FIGURE 10: Example of a goal/excuse card

Carry your index card with you for the next week. Whenever you think about performing your goal, especially if you don't really feel like doing it, pull the card out and read both sides. Ask yourself, "Can I do this anyway, even though my mind is giving me lots of excuses not to?" The key is to recognize that you can carry your excuses with you but you don't have to obey them—you can have those words show up inside your head *and* simultaneously carry out some health-promoting action.

You can use this system whenever you start work on a new health goal. Be warned, though. The moment you start striving for your goals, you'll also increase your rate of failure. This is true for all goal striving. The chapter on kind motivation (Chapter 9) will help prepare you for setbacks and show you how to develop lasting motivation.

The flexible mindset

Once we stop clinging so tightly to rigid diet rules (and our reasons for breaking them), we can start being more flexible. We don't *have to* slavishly follow the diet rules. Nor do we have to generate excuses for not having a healthy lifestyle. We're more flexible and can respond to what our body actually needs. The flexible mindset allows us to persist with behaviors that are working for us, and to change behaviors that aren't working. In the rest of this book we'll work on developing this flexible mindset. For now, here are a few signs that indicate a more flexible, less rigid diet mindset:

- Awareness of what you're eating.
- Awareness of your motivation for eating (e.g., boredom, stress, anxiety, trying to cheer yourself up).
- Reminding yourself "If I eat too much on one day, I can eat a little less on the next day."
- When it comes to eating a favorite high-calorie treat, practicing portion control, eating it slowly and savoring it rather than forbidding yourself from ever eating it.
- Adopting a more-or-less approach to exercise, rather than slavishly obeying an all-or-nothing rule. For example, if you don't have time to exercise for 50 minutes at the gym, as you intended, then exercise for 20 minutes instead, or go for a 10-minute walk, whatever your timetable permits.

STOP!

Your mind will probably try to talk you out of letting go of diet rules. Stop for a moment and listen in. Can you hear it saying things like "This won't work! How can I possibly lose weight without strict rules? If I don't follow the rules I'll pig out and stuff myself." The good news is, you don't have to listen to what your mind says. As we found in the previous chapter, the mind is an unreliable adviser. Instead of clinging to rigid rules, you can develop flexible dieting principles like those outlined below.

SIX FLEXIBLE DIETING PRINCIPLES

These principles don't require you to follow a specific diet plan that emphasizes, for example, protein or carbohydrates or fat. We leave the choice of diet plan up to you and your preferences. The six principles don't require you to eat foods you dislike or to deprive yourself. These principles are based on the best possible scientific evidence, and indicate ways you can safely lose weight while also increasing your energy, health and wellbeing.

The key to using the six principles is flexibility: you'll need to ignore, or go against them, many times. To encourage you to be flexible, we've ended each principle with a flexibility reminder. These reminders will emphasize exceptions to the principles, and show that no principle can or should be followed all the time.

Whatever sort of diet you choose, you'll probably make use of most, if not all, of the six diet principles. Indeed, if you follow one of the principles, you'll tend to follow them all, because they're interrelated. For example, eating a lot of fruit and vegetables (Principle 5) will lower the energy density of your diet (Principle 2), lower its glycemic index (Principle 3) and increase its nutritional density (Principle 4).

1. The key to weight loss is energy deficit without deprivation

Energy deficit occurs when you burn more calories than you consume. You can do this by doing more exercise and/or decreasing your calorie intake. If you've ever lost weight, it was because you went into energy deficit. There's no other magical way to lose weight, and any diet plan that tells you otherwise is lying. There are three things you can do to create energy deficit:

- Reduce portion size of meals and snacks. This often involves eating fewer servings of high-calorie food, especially those foods with little nutritional value (see appendix for guide to serving sizes).
- Decrease energy density of food (see below).
- Increase activity.

It is important to remember that going into energy deficit doesn't mean you have to go into life deficit. You don't have to give up the things you love. The key is to practice portion control and to think in terms of eating *more* of the right food. The next four principles will help you target the quality, rather than quantity, of your food. Improving the quality of your diet will lead to healthy weight loss without you feeling hungry all the time, or irritable or fatigued. A quality diet leads to a life of sustained energy and health.

Flexibility reminder: It would be impossible to be in energy deficit all the time. Sometimes you'll choose to go into energy surplus and eat "too much." You might want to enjoy a feast with your family and friends, for example. There's no need for you to be on a perfect diet. Rather, the key is to make changes to your lifestyle that will help you to sustain a healthy weight over time.

2. The secret to eating satisfying amounts of food and losing weight is energy density

Foods with a high energy density give you a lot of calories in a small quantity. They don't fill you up. These foods include many sweets and cakes, fatty meat and white bread. In contrast, foods with a low energy density have a lot of weight and fill you up, but don't give you a lot of calories. Such foods include vegetables, fruit, salads and most soups, among other things. The more water in the food, the lower its energy density, so for example grapes have lower energy density than raisins. The energy-dense foods take up little space in the stomach, whereas the low-density food fills the stomach and is satisfying.

You can decrease the energy density of your food without depriving yourself. For example, if you focus on increasing your intake of vegetables, healthy soups and salads while reducing the amount of high-density foods like fries, you can eat just as much food without consuming so many calories. You can also replace high-density ingredients with low-density alternatives. If you use a pound of ground beef in your pasta, you can change this to 12 ounces and make up the difference with puréed vegetables. The amazing thing is that adding puréed vegetables doesn't alter the taste of the food. If you're interested in exploring energy-density diets in more detail, we strongly recommend the book *The Ultimate Volumetrics Diet* by Barbara Rolls. We're hesitant to recommend any diet book, but Barbara Rolls is one of the best regarded and most rigorous nutritionists in the field, and we feel confident in her work. We have also placed some energy density tables in the appendix, and some instruction on how you can calculate energy density for yourself.

Flexibility reminder: Some energy-dense foods, such as nuts and cheese, can be good for you in moderation.

ENERGY DENSITY: KEY PRINCIPLES

- Swap. Practice swapping higher energy-dense foods for lower energy-dense foods. This allows you to eat the same number of servings of food each day but reduces the number of calories you eat.
- Don't deprive yourself. Your diet should not leave you feeling hungry. Find ways to eat larger amounts of low energy-dense foods (see appendix).
- Eat more fruits, vegetables, and other low-density foods.
- Cook smart. When cooking, reduce high-fat ingredients, increase water-rich ingredients. For example, add vegetables to main dishes like omelettes, lasagne, pizza, chili, soups and other hot dishes.
- Become aware of the energy density in aspects of your diet and portion sizes (see appendix).

3. The secret to sustained energy is food with a low glycemic index

Foods with a *high* glycemic index (GI)—such as white rice, doughnuts, white bread, soft drinks and sugary cereals—give a rapid but short-lived burst of energy. If you eat a lot of these foods, your energy levels are likely to become highly variable, and when your energy suddenly drops, you tend to seek out a quick hit of sugary food. In contrast, foods with a low GI—such as brown rice, cherries, most legumes, multigrain bread and some bran-based cereals—allow you to sustain your energy over time. If you eat a lot of high-GI food, it might be a good idea to find ways to eat less of it. Lower-GI diets are associated with a lower risk of cardiovascular disease, better metabolic function and successful weight loss. (See appendix for a guide to the GI of many common foods.)

Flexibility reminder: Some low-GI foods may not have high nutritional value or may contain substantial fat. A typical mass-market chocolate bar, for example, has a low GI, but that doesn't make it healthy—it's loaded with fat and sugar and is very high in calories. At the same time, some high-GI foods can be good for you due to the other nutrients they contain, such as pumpkin.

4. The secret to protecting yourself from disease is nutritional density

You can think of nutritional density as the amount of bang you get for your calorie buck. Something with a high nutritional density has a high proportion of nutrients to calories. Examples of nutrient-dense foods include vegetables, fruit, legumes and raw nuts and seeds. Foods with low nutritional density include red meat, cheese, cookies, cakes, candy and soft drinks. Plant-based foods tend to be highest in nutritional density, as they contain many vitamins, minerals and other health-promoting substances.

Increasing the nutritional density of your food will be likely to improve your health, promote weight loss and reduce your risk of cancer, heart disease, stroke and Alzheimer's disease. One interesting study suggests that increasing nutritional density might even change how you experience hunger. People who shift from a low-nutrient-density to a high-nutrient-density diet may initially experience an unpleasant withdrawal from unhealthy foods, but over time, as their body adjusts to the healthier diet, they'll experience hunger as less unpleasant.

Flexibility reminder: Foods can be classified as low in nutritional density but nevertheless be healthy. For example, meat tends to be less nutrient-dense than plant foods. Nevertheless, if you're not a vegetarian, meat can be a healthy part of your diet. Lean red meat can be a valuable source of iron and protein, and fish can be a good source of healthy omega-3 fatty acids.

5. Whole foods are better than processed foods and supplements

Regular consumption of whole foods such as fruit and vegetables is associated with reduced risk of cancer, cardiovascular disease, stroke, Alzheimer's disease and cataracts. When researchers first made this discovery, they set about trying to extract the key nutrients from fruit and vegetables, the "magic bullet" that would prevent disease. They wondered if vitamin E could prevent cancer, or vitamin C could prevent the common cold.

Unfortunately, after years of work, these researchers were unable to show that the extracted nutrients provided the same benefit as the whole food. It turned out you had to eat an actual orange to get the benefit, rather than consuming lots of vitamin C extracted from the orange. Or to take another example, your risk of cancer is reduced if you eat a lot of green and yellow vegetables and fruit, which contain beta-carotene, but ingesting beta-carotene as a supplement has either no effect, or actually increases the risk of cancer and in rare cases, even death.

Whole foods contain many nutrients and other substances in combinations that have not been recreated in supplement form. For example, there are thousands of different natural chemicals in plants that help those plants defend themselves against environmental threats such as pests. It turns out these chemicals may protect humans as well. But while they may provide some benefit on their own, their effect is largely due to them working together with other food chemicals. To summarize, whatever diet you choose, you should make sure it includes many whole foods and few processed foods, and doesn't depend on supplements.

Flexibility reminder: There may be instances where whole foods are not readily available, or where a health professional recommends a meal replacement drink in the context of an otherwise healthy diet. There may also be instances where supplements are useful, such as when recommended by a doctor to treat a vitamin deficiency.

6. Don't deprive yourself—swap!

So many diets require you to give up things, such as carbs or fat or sweets. But it's not much fun going through life feeling deprived.

Instead, we recommend a "swap" mentality. Instead of getting rid of "bad" foods, think in terms of *improving* your diet by swapping less healthy foods for more healthy ones. The table below gives some examples.

RECOMMENDED FOOD SWAPS

SWAP THIS	FOR THIS
Regular beer	Low-calorie beer
Whole milk	Low-fat milk
Regular latte	Skinny latte
Creamy, cheesy pasta sauce	Tomato-based pasta sauce
Fatty meat	Lean meat
A large piece of meat	A small piece of meat with lots of vegetables
Soft drink	Tea or sparkling water
Deep-fried fast food	Fresh fast food (grilled fish and salad, sandwiches with lean meats and lots of vegetables or salad)
Cake or other high-calorie dessert	Yogurt and fruit

Flexibility reminder: Sometimes you'll want to do a "reverse swap," where you decide, for example, to have an indulgent dessert instead of a bowl of fruit. Expect every principle to be broken occasionally. Of course, when you do a reverse swap, it's better to choose a small portion size and eat it slowly, truly savoring it.

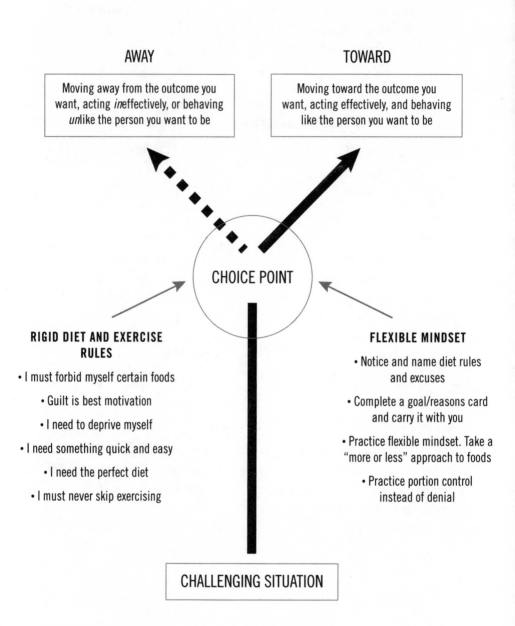

FIGURE 11: Practice flexibility

SUMMARY: IF YOU WISH TO LOSE WEIGHT . . .

DO MORE OF THIS	DO LESS OF THIS
Defuse from rigid diet rules.	Fuse with (be dominated by) rigid diet rules. Sacrifice everything in order to lose the weight.
Take a more-or-less approach. Allow yourself to have some indulgent treats but practice portion control.	Take an all-or-nothing approach. Forbid yourself to eat foods you love. Believe yourself a failure if you eat anything you're "not supposed to."
Recognize that the mind is skillful at creating reasons for not doing things. Learn to notice these reasons without letting them dominate your behavior.	Let reason-giving rule your life.
Use the six flexible diet principles to help create a diet that suits your personal tastes and interests.	Keep searching for the perfect diet, or the quick and easy trick. Go on a diet that's completely unsuited to your tastes and lifestyle.

6.
LISTENING TO YOUR BODY

How long have we been at war with our bodies? We hate the parts of ourselves that are "too big" and seek to destroy them with sit-ups or squats. Hunger is seen as a powerful enemy that, at any moment, may overwhelm our defenses. Cravings are like dangerous soldiers, hiding in the bushes, waiting to spring the trap, and when they've captured us, they'll force us to eat that supersized block of chocolate. We've fought against cravings, resisted urges and battled hunger with all our might— and almost always, we've been ground down and defeated.

But you know, deep down, this war is futile. You can see it hasn't been working for you in the long term. And that's only to be expected. The internal war doesn't work for anybody. It didn't work for any of us, the authors, and it certainly hasn't worked for any of our clients, friends or family members. Why not?

Because that urge, craving or feeling you struggle with is a part of you. It's just as much a part of you as your hands and feet, your eyes and ears. How can fighting with parts of yourself ever lead to something good? It's just tiring, stressful and ultimately demoralizing. And it only gives more energy to the "I'm not good enough" story (see Chapter 4).

So are you ready to broker a peace treaty with your body? If yes, then you're ready to tackle a new challenge: namely, to build a new alliance between mind and body. For most of us, our mind and our body are strangers to each other. It's time for us to set that straight.

NON-HUNGRY EATING

Most of us live inside our head. We get so caught up inside our thoughts, we lose touch with our body. Unfortunately, the more disconnected we are from our body, the more we lose touch with our healthy hunger signals. And then we really get into trouble.

We start eating for reasons that have nothing to do with genuine hunger. Rather, we eat because we crave sugar or fat (see "Distinguishing Hunger from a Craving" on page 115), or we feel stressed or lonely. We eat out of boredom, or to distract ourselves. We eat on automatic pilot, simply because the food is there in front of us. We eat to rebel against an unfair society that demands we be unreasonably thin. We eat out of habit, or to please the person who's provided the food, or simply to follow the rule that we can't leave a plate until it's empty.

In short, we engage in a lot of *non-hungry eating*. Non-hungry eating is a major cause of weight gain, because we consume far more calories than our body needs. In this chapter, we'll help you recognize the difference between non-hungry and hungry eating.

To lose weight and keep it off, we need to cut down on non-hungry eating. Notice that we use the words "cut down" rather than "cut out." We don't want your mind to create a new commandment for you: "Thou shalt never practice non-hungry eating." Non-hungry eating is neither bad nor good, in and of itself. Our aim is to make non-hungry eating a conscious choice rather than your default setting.

This whole book is ultimately about helping you have more choices in life. We only want you to eat less if that's what you consciously choose to do, from a space of mental flexibility not rigidity. There are times when it can be joyful to choose to engage in non-hungry eating, such as when celebrating with loved ones. At other times, however, we may choose to avoid non-hungry eating, such as when the food isn't very tasty or healthy, or when we want to give our weight-loss goals priority.

The only way we'll get to choose is to become aware of our hunger signals with the skills described in the right side of the figure opposite. Without such awareness, our impulses, cravings, urges, feelings and sensations will push us to eat, even when we're not hungry. The good news is our bodies have a wisdom we can learn to hear.

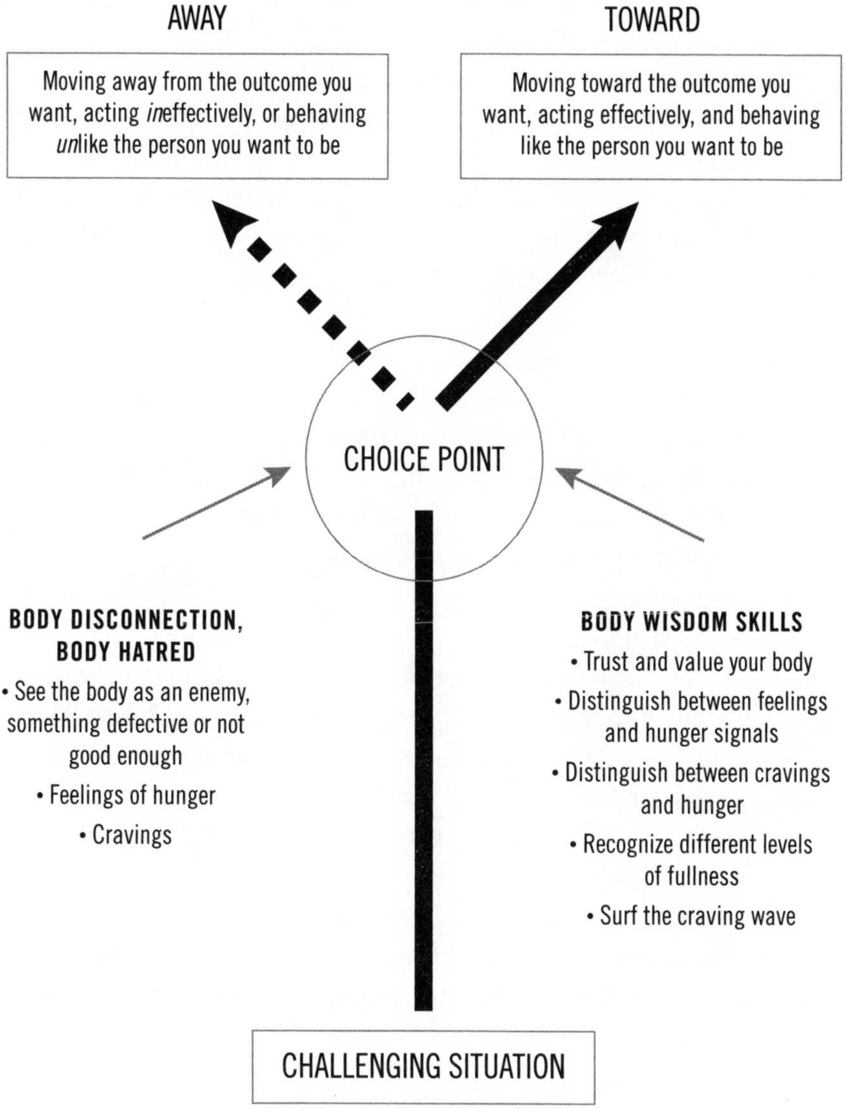

AWAY

TOWARD

Moving away from the outcome you want, acting *in*effectively, or behaving *un*like the person you want to be

Moving toward the outcome you want, acting effectively, and behaving like the person you want to be

CHOICE POINT

BODY DISCONNECTION, BODY HATRED

- See the body as an enemy, something defective or not good enough
  - Feelings of hunger
    - Cravings

BODY WISDOM SKILLS

- Trust and value your body
- Distinguish between feelings and hunger signals
- Distinguish between cravings and hunger
- Recognize different levels of fullness
- Surf the craving wave

CHALLENGING SITUATION

FIGURE 12: Awareness and recognition of hunger signals help us make better food choices

EXERCISE: **AM I REALLY HUNGRY?**

Hunger signals vary enormously for each of us. We might experience them in our abdomen, throat or mouth; they might be moving or still, mild or intense. This exercise will help you become more aware of your hunger signals, so you can learn to differentiate them from cravings, urges, anxiety and other unpleasant emotions. This will give you greater freedom and choice. It's best to do this exercise when you're feeling hungry, ideally after delaying your lunch or dinner. Please don't rush it; at least the first time you do it, spend 10–15 seconds on each step. There are no right answers—the questions are just an aid to the exercise of noticing and listening to your body when it is hungry.

1. **Notice your breath**
   When you are hungry, sit quietly, in a comfortable position, and turn your attention to your breath. Breathe in, pause, and breathe out. Notice the flow of the breath in and out of your nostrils. Observe your breath with curiosity. You don't have to change your breathing, just let it be. If thoughts distract you, just notice those thoughts with curiosity.

2. **Notice your mouth**
   Notice any sensations you might be experiencing inside your mouth. What do you notice inside your cheeks, in your gums, teeth and jaws? Can you notice any increase in temperature or saliva building up as you search for the sensations of hunger?

3. **Notice your tongue**
   What do you notice on your tongue? Do you feel hunger here? Are there any tingling or prickling sensations? Or perhaps an increase in temperature? Where are these sensations? On the front of your tongue, the sides or back?

4. **Notice your throat**
   What hunger sensations do you notice in your throat? Is it dry or moist? Tight or loose? Do you notice any urge to swallow? Or perhaps a sense of thirst?

5. **Notice your stomach**
   Are there any hunger sensations in your stomach? Is there any sense of hollowness or emptiness? Any rumbling or gurgling? Twisting or turning? Can

you tell if it's full or empty or somewhere in between? Is there any tightness, tingling or perhaps even mild nausea? And whereabouts in your abdomen are these sensations most intense: at the top, near the ribcage, right in the middle, behind the belly button, or around the sides?

6. **Notice your head**

    How does your head feel? Light or heavy? Achy or dizzy? Do you feel fatigued, energetic, agitated or edgy? Do you feel any pressure or tension in your forehead?

7. **Reflect: is this hunger?**

    Now consider: which of these sensations are most familiar to you? Are these feelings in your mouth, tongue, throat, stomach and head typical of what you feel when you're truly hungry? Can you distinguish these feelings and sensations from cravings for comfort food high in sugar and fat, unpleasant emotions like anxiety or sadness, or urges to treat yourself or indulge your tastebuds?

    If you can't distinguish your genuine hunger from emotional cues to eat, you'll need to do more practice; repeat this exercise as many times as you have to until you can distinguish hunger from other triggers to eat. If you can clearly recognize these feelings as hunger, then say to yourself whenever you feel them: "Here's hunger" or "I'm noticing hunger."

8. **Notice your mind**

    Finally, notice what your mind is saying to you right now. Is it telling you to eat something, quickly? Is it generating pictures of tasty foods or figuring out what your eating options are? Is it judging these feelings as bad or unbearable in some way, and telling you you need to get rid of them as soon as possible?

We recommend you practice this hunger meditation at least once a day for a full week. But like any skill, the more you practice, the better. If you can do it two or three times a day, fantastic!

Many people initially find it hard to distinguish genuine hunger from other triggers to eat, such as anxiety, sadness, loneliness, boredom or cravings for fat and sugar. In order to connect with and recognize your hunger cues effectively, you'll need to manipulate your meal times so that you're more likely to experience genuine hunger. If it's possible, therefore, push back lunch or dinner regularly, and complete steps 1–8. It will help you begin to identify the physical cues that signal genuine hunger and recognize better when the cues to eat are not hunger.

Whenever you feel the desire to eat, pause for a moment, take a slow breath, and scan your body as in steps 1–8 above, noting the sensations in your mouth, cheeks, jaws, tongue, throat and stomach. With practice, you can easily do this in five to 10 seconds. Then ask yourself two questions: "Is my stomach genuinely hungry, or is it just my mouth wanting flavor? Is my stomach genuinely hungry, or am I trying to comfort myself with food?" Finally, remind yourself "If I truly want to eat it, I can. The choice is mine. But do I really want to put this into my body?'

Understanding how hungry you are

Now that we've done the fundamental work of understanding hunger cues, we'll take our sensitivity to the next level by understanding the stages of hunger. The Levels of Hunger scale below will help you to discern how hungry or full you are at any given moment. Let's take a moment to practice using this scale right now.

LEVELS OF HUNGER

Rate your hunger right now according to the hunger scale below.

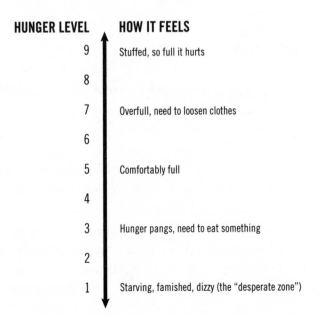

HUNGER LEVEL	HOW IT FEELS
9	Stuffed, so full it hurts
8	
7	Overfull, need to loosen clothes
6	
5	Comfortably full
4	
3	Hunger pangs, need to eat something
2	
1	Starving, famished, dizzy (the "desperate zone")

The Levels of Hunger scale will help you notice different body states. Learn to eat when you're around 3 on this scale. Listen to your body. Don't wait until you're completely famished to eat or there's a good chance that out of desperation you'll eat something extremely unhealthy or eat far more than you need, or both.

It takes a good 10–15 minutes for the signal of stomach fullness to reach the satiety centers in the brain; only once the brain receives these signals will you feel comfortably full. Because of this time delay, it's a good idea to stop eating *before* you feel full. So, for example, if you stop eating when it feels like you're on level 5, you'll probably actually end up on level 6. It might be best to stop eating at around level 4 then wait to see what your body tells you. If you're still hungry after 10–15 minutes, you might choose to eat some more.

Distinguishing hunger from a craving

Hunger tells us what our bodies *need* whereas cravings tell us what our bodies *want*. We eventually have to eat if we're hungry, but we don't have to eat when we have a craving. Indulging a craving is a form of non-hungry eating. If you want to cut down on calories and lose weight, it makes sense to cut down on the extent you eat by listening to cravings.

By learning to recognize a craving, we allow ourselves an important moment of choice with several options available:

- We can let the craving come and go, in its own good time, without indulging it, in the service of taking care of ourselves.
- We can indulge the craving in moderation.
- We can indulge the craving without restraint.

But if we want this freedom of choice, we must first learn to recognize the craving when it arises, so that we don't go on automatic pilot and start eating before we even realize what we're doing.

Hunger is driven by our body's physical needs. Cravings are usually driven by environmental factors, such as the sight or smell of food, or psychological factors, such as unpleasant feelings and emotions. The table below illustrates some of the key differences between hunger and cravings.

HUNGER VERSUS A CRAVING

HUNGER	CRAVING
Driven by the body's needs	Triggered by psychological or environmental factors (e.g., stress, the sight of chocolate)
Doesn't go away if you wait it out	Often goes away if you wait it out
Intensifies over time	Doesn't intensify over time
Can only be taken away by eating	Can be taken away by doing something else (e.g., engaging in a valued activity)
Can be alleviated by almost any food	Can be alleviated by only one food

EMOTIONAL EATING

A craving often involves the desire to get rid of an emotion by eating something specific like chocolate. Food momentarily gives us relief from emotional pain: it distracts us, soothes us or helps us zone out. When we satisfy a craving through food, it can feel very similar to satisfying our hunger with food. No wonder we get confused! The only ways we can break through this confusion are by increasing our awareness of genuine hunger and improving our ability to distinguish it from a craving.

This quick exercise will help you get better at recognizing a craving.

EXERCISE: SPOTTING THE CRAVING

Take a moment to remember a time you really craved something (e.g., chocolate, chips, ice cream, pizza). Really bring that memory to mind. How were you feeling? What were you thinking?

Now get in touch with your craving by describing it as a physical object. If your craving had a shape, what would it be (e.g., a box, a spear)? If your craving had a color, what would it be? If your craving had a temperature, how hot or cold would it be? If your craving had a texture, how would it feel?

The next step to building awareness is to monitor your cravings, that is, when and where you feel a strong desire to eat a specific food. One great way to do this is to keep a craving journal, noting your cravings each day and analyzing your emotional state each time. This will help you build awareness of your cravings over time and strengthen your ability to resist them when you want to. For more, see "Keeping a Craving Journal" opposite.

EXERCISE: **KEEPING A CRAVING JOURNAL**

The form below will make it easier to identify your craving triggers. To start with, fill it out for a few days, to practice awareness of when you have strong desires for a specific food. Notice each time when your desire for a specific food was driven by physical hunger, and when it was not. Also notice if your cravings occur regularly at a particular time of day.

DATE AND TIME	FOOD CRAVED	PLACE CRAVING OCCURRED	HOW THE CRAVING FELT	RATING (1–9) ON HUNGER SCALE	RESULT (1 = DIDN'T GIVE IN, 9 = GAVE IN COMPLETELY)

After a few days of keeping your journal, analyze the results. Do you have a regular craving for a particular food or at a particular time of day? Does a particular emotional state trigger your cravings? Did the cravings become easier to resist as your awareness of them developed?

RIDING THE CRAVING WAVE

The good news is that cravings, unlike hunger, will pass with time, even if you don't eat anything. A craving is like a wave. It's neither good nor bad. Imagine for a moment a wave beginning to form. Imagine it starts small and grows slowly, gathering momentum and reaching a peak in size and power. Finally it crashes down on the beach. Think about how hard it would be to stop that wave. The power of the wave is so great, if you get in its way, it will slam against you or dunk you.

Like a wave, a craving starts off small, builds to a peak and then passes. But we rarely let a craving reach its peak, because as it builds up it feels more and more unpleasant and humans don't particularly like unpleasant feelings.

Unfortunately, the fastest way to get rid of any urge or craving is to indulge it—which means, once again, we're back to non-hungry eating. But there's an alternative way to handle our urges and cravings. Instead of fighting them, we can learn to ride them out; we can surf the craving, just as we might surf a wave. To learn how, try the following exercise.

EXERCISE: **URGE SURFING**

Next time you feel the urge to eat something (i.e., a craving) and you don't really want to eat it because you're not hungry, try the following.

1. **Pause and breathe**

   When a craving shows up, your mind will tell you that you need to act fast: "Eat now or you'll die of misery!" your mind will insist. So the first step in dealing with the craving is to slow down.

   Take five long, slow, deep breaths. Notice the breath flowing into your lungs. And notice it exiting again. There's no need to rush anything. You can make your choice later. Just notice your breath and slow yourself down.

2. **Notice and name**

   Next, notice the urge. Where is it located? In your stomach? In your mouth? In your head? Watch with curiosity as the urge develops and changes, as if you were a child observing an amazing event. Give your urge a name. For example, you might say, "Here comes the chocolate wave." Or you might just say to yourself, "I notice I'm having an urge." Or simply, "Craving!"

3. **Choose**

   Now that you've paused and noticed the urge, you're ready to choose your action. You can either indulge the urge or you can surf it. The choice is yours.

Note: this is very different from resisting an urge; here we're making space for the craving, allowing it to come and stay and go in its own good time and taking conscious control of what we do while the craving is present.

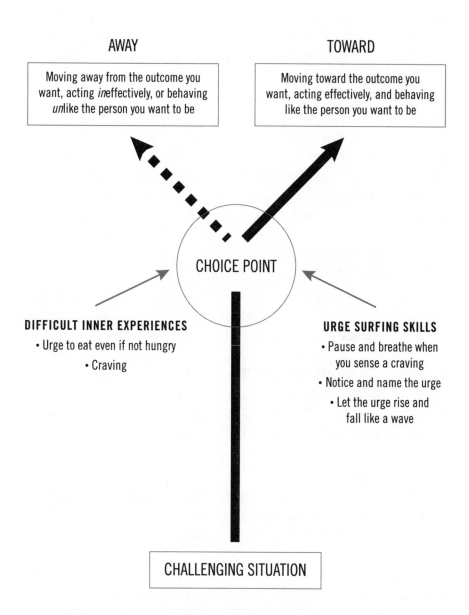

FIGURE 13: Making space for the urge allows you to surf it

Developing a craving plan

Surfing your cravings and urges will require practice. Sometimes the craving will catch you off guard and you'll indulge it before you even realize it. Indeed, we can say this with 100 percent certainty: you'll sometimes be ruled by your cravings. Everybody experiences this. Strength of character can't be measured by whether or not we indulge or surf our cravings. It's measured by our willingness to recommit to our health goals, over and over and over again, no matter how many times we go off-track.

You can make it easier to ride the waves of craving by creating a plan of action. This *craving plan* will help you anticipate times when cravings will be fierce and allow you to develop a health-enhancing action as an alternative to indulging the craving. We recommend you develop your own individualized craving plan based on the following three steps.

1. REMOVE OR AVOID THE THINGS THAT TRIGGER YOUR CRAVINGS

For example, if you crave chocolate, chips or ice cream and you don't want to eat much of these things, it would be a good idea not to have them in the house.

2. DO SOMETHING YOU CARE ABOUT INSTEAD OF INDULGING THE CRAVING

For example, you might call a friend, listen to music, exercise or play a game. You can deliberately choose to engage in a valued activity and say to yourself, "This is what I choose to do."

3. INDULGE YOURSELF *A LITTLE* AT TIMES

Do this especially if the craving is something you do for the pleasure of it and not just to avoid or get rid of unpleasant feelings. In the next chapter, you'll learn how to indulge mindfully.

Take a moment to plan for your craving by answering the questions below. Remind yourself that if you've read this far and are consciously thinking about how to manage your cravings, you've already taken a big step.

- What can I do to avoid the things that trigger my craving?
- What other fun or interesting activity can I do instead of indulging the craving?

SUMMARY: IF YOU WISH TO LOSE WEIGHT . . .

DO MORE OF THIS	DO LESS OF THIS
Listen to your body and recognize when it's hungry.	Ignore your body. Fight it with fad diets that leave you starving and deprived.
Become aware of your hunger level and pause in your eating when you're comfortably full.	Ignore your hunger cues and eat until you're overfull or so stuffed it hurts.
Recognize the difference between hunger and cravings.	React as if cravings mean you *have* to eat.
Practice riding the craving wave. Create your individualized craving plan.	Always give in to craving waves before they reach their peak.

PART I SUMMARY

In the first part of this book we have talked about how we often respond ineffectually to challenging situations and difficult inner experiences. We often do things such as emotional eating or trying to stick to rigid diet rules that take us away from what we want. The good news is that neither the situation nor our inner experiences force us to act ineffectually. We can learn to respond to challenging situations with a mindful pause—that brief moment of time we need in order to step back and choose. It is in that pause that we will find our freedom. Figure 14 summarizes all the skills we have learned so far.

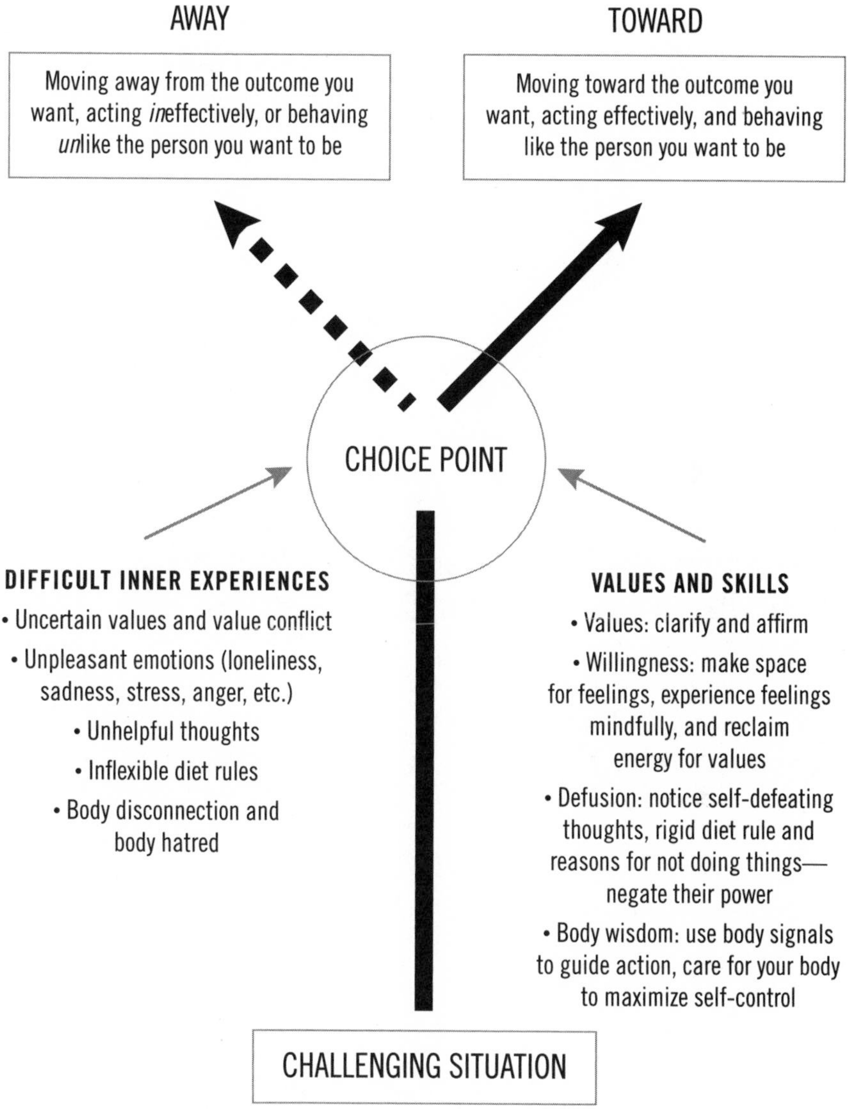

AWAY

Moving away from the outcome you want, acting *in*effectively, or behaving *un*like the person you want to be

TOWARD

Moving toward the outcome you want, acting effectively, and behaving like the person you want to be

CHOICE POINT

DIFFICULT INNER EXPERIENCES

• Uncertain values and value conflict

• Unpleasant emotions (loneliness, sadness, stress, anger, etc.)

• Unhelpful thoughts

• Inflexible diet rules

• Body disconnection and body hatred

VALUES AND SKILLS

• Values: clarify and affirm

• Willingness: make space for feelings, experience feelings mindfully, and reclaim energy for values

• Defusion: notice self-defeating thoughts, rigid diet rule and reasons for not doing things— negate their power

• Body wisdom: use body signals to guide action, care for your body to maximize self-control

CHALLENGING SITUATION

FIGURE 14: Summary of skills involved in the Choice Point model

PART 2:

BUILDING A NEW LIFE

7.
DEVELOPING THE MINDFULNESS HABIT

LOST TIME, MISSED OPPORTUNITIES

"I've got to get out the door as soon as possible," Lisa thinks. "I have too many things to do." Lisa yells at her daughter to hurry up. She seems to go slow on purpose. Then Lisa yells "Get dressed," and leaves the room to get herself ready for work. She comes back out and the girl is still not ready and she yells at her again. Then she yells "Eat your breakfast now, we have to get going." Lisa rushes to the computer to send a few emails. She comes back out and tells the girl, "Let's go. Quickly. We are going to be late!"

That night, Lisa discovers a crayon drawing on the table from that morning. It shows a mother and daughter with smiles on their faces, and a sun shining in the background. Underneath is written, "I love my mom."

That same day, John drives quickly to work, carefully avoiding the speed traps. He curses his bad luck for having a meeting that day with Jessica about some stupid health and safety policy. He already has too much to do. When Jessica comes for the meeting, his body surges with stress and his mind keeps reminding him of all he has to do. He answers her questions tersely and after 20 minutes, he abruptly ends the meeting.

Later that day, John is talking to his friend who says, "Did you hear about Jessica? Her husband has been diagnosed with cancer. It's bad. He probably won't make it."

We struggle to stay in the present moment. We often eat without noticing, talk to others without really listening to them and rush through the day as if it's one long list of chores to be crossed off our list before time runs out.

We humans seem restless and lost compared with other animals. Imagine you and a dog are both at a public park, for example, and it's just rained. The dog sits on the wet grass and feels the sun warming his back. That's all he seems to need in that moment. We can sit there too, but our minds are likely to be judging everything: "I don't have time to just sit here. I've got work to do. Is the grass too wet? Are my clothes getting dirty? Will those ants crawl on my skin?"

Our words create a world inside our head and we get stuck there. Our eyes become closed to the physical world. We feel swept away, like we're dreaming and unable to control what we do and what happens next. In brief moments, we recognize that we're dreaming and we struggle to wake up.

The first part of this book began the process of increasing our awareness. Specifically, we've become more aware of the following:

1. How we all seek to reduce our suffering by fighting our feelings and thoughts, and how this often backfires to make our suffering worse (Chapters 2 and 3).
2. How our minds are judgmental and fallible, and never stop offering us advice. Once we become aware of that advice, we're free to follow it or ignore it (Chapters 4 and 5).
3. How we often declare war on our bodies. Then we can learn to make peace with ourselves and become aware of the wisdom of our bodies (Chapter 6).

The truth is, awareness comes and goes. We get stressed, we get busy, we get upset—and just like that, our awareness flies out the window, we switch to automatic pilot and we forget about our values and our commitments. So we need to prepare ourselves for those challenging times—for those tough moments of stress, anxiety and pressure—so we can remain aware in the midst of our distress and stick to our own core values. In other words, we need to make awareness into a habit by developing the *mindfulness* habit. *Mindfulness* means paying attention, with an attitude of openness and curiosity.

GOOD AND BAD HABITS

A habit is a pattern of behavior that we've repeated so often that it becomes natural and easy to do. Everyone has "bad" habits. By bad we don't mean morally wrong, we just mean that instead of enriching and enhancing life, these habits make it worse. And when it comes to eating, most of us have been the victim of at least a few bad habits. You might have got into the habit of stopping at a fast-food place while driving home, for example, or eating something loaded with sugar and fat after dinner, or drinking mindlessly and munching on snacks while vegging in front of the TV immediately after work. Or maybe you have a habit of finishing all the food on your plate, even when you're not hungry.

Habits happen fairly automatically and unconsciously. Even small bad eating habits can lead to weight gain. The simple habit of eating a cookie or muffin with morning tea, for example, can add pounds of fat to your body over the course of a year. At the same time, swapping one good habit for one bad habit can lead to lasting weight loss. If, for example, we cut 350 calories per day by eating a salad instead of a high-calorie lunch, we'll lose about 10 pounds within four months. And that's from just one habit change!

The great thing about developing a good eating habit is that it can help us keep making healthy eating choices without requiring us to constantly use willpower or self-discipline. Suppose you make a habit of eating a healthy lunch, for example. It will take time, but once the habit is entrenched, you'll be able to shop for, make and eat such lunches without thinking about it. If you can make exercise into a routine, you might eventually find it harder to break the routine than to keep it. Your body will cry out for exercise.

Building new habits: the key to lasting change

Habits begin with a simple cue, followed by an immediate reward. We see the vending machine just before lunch when we're hungry (the cue), and then we buy the potato chips and eat them (the reward). If we do that often enough, we develop a *habit loop* (see Figure 15 below): when we see the cue, we automatically go into a chip-buying routine. We don't even think about whether it's a good idea for our health or whether we really want chips.

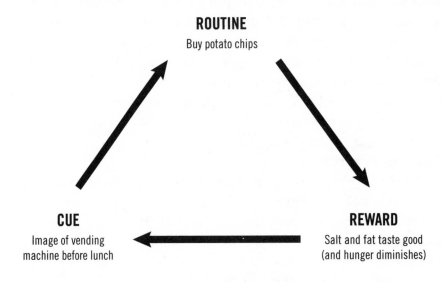

ROUTINE
Buy potato chips

CUE
Image of vending
machine before lunch

REWARD
Salt and fat taste good
(and hunger diminishes)

FIGURE 15: The habit loop

Something very interesting happens in our brain as habits form. Initially, our brain generates a pleasure response only *after* we receive the actual reward. So, in the example above, our brain only lights up with pleasure after we eat the potato chips. As the habit loop is practiced and practiced, however, (as we regularly stop at the vending machine to buy chips), something changes. The brain's pleasure response starts to occur *before* we actually receive the reward; the cue alone is enough to trigger it. In other words, we start to experience pleasure the moment we see the vending machine; we learn to expect the reward. Indeed, even thinking about the vending machine can be enough to trigger the pleasure.

So what happens the day we go on a diet and decide to bypass the vending machine? If the habit loop has been established and we walk by the machine without buying the chips, our body will react with a pleasure response. But then, when we don't engage in our normal routine (buying the chips), we'll experience a craving. We'll feel pushed toward the machine. We'll feel tense or disappointed if we don't buy the chips.

Before we developed a habit loop, we might not even have noticed the machine there, but now it pulls at us like an industrial magnet. You can begin to see how detrimental this can be; habit can become a force that pulls us in an unhelpful direction. But the flip side is that the habit can actually pull us in a helpful direction. Imagine if our habitual exercise program actively pulls us in to engage with it, even when we don't feel in the mood. Or if our habit of healthy eating pulls us in to make a healthy choice in the midst of a smorgasbord of temptation.

So how do we make the force of habit work for us instead of against us? We start by developing what we call the *ultimate habit*. It will be the most important habit you'll learn because it will be the habit that helps you break other habits. This foundational habit upon which most other good habits will rest is called *mindfulness*.

Why mindfulness is essential

When we perform any activity mindfully, we get far more out of it, because as we pay attention, with openness and curiosity, we become increasingly engaged in it. When we eat mindfully, we consciously choose our food; we eat intentionally, to serve a life-enhancing purpose; and we savor what we eat, noticing the taste, texture and sheer pleasure, thereby maximizing our satisfaction and fulfillment. This is the very opposite of eating *mindlessly*—putting food into our mouth on automatic pilot, without consciously choosing what or how much we'll consume or taking the time to truly savor it. It's not hard to see how *mindless eating* readily leads to weight gain and *mindful eating* reverses it.

The great thing about developing the mindfulness habit is that you can do it any time, anywhere, for as little or as long as you like. One way to develop our capacity for mindfulness is by taking up ancient Eastern practices such as yoga, meditation, Tai Chi or martial arts.

Another is by bringing mindfulness to bear on our everyday activities, so that we engage in mindful walking, mindful cooking, mindful cleaning, mindful exercising, mindful driving, mindful parenting or mindful conversations.

The benefits of mindfulness

Mindfulness puts you, rather than your impulses, in charge. We all have the potential to act impulsively. That doesn't mean there's something wrong with us. Impulsiveness can be useful in many situations, especially when we have to make rapid life or death choices. Imagine a hungry tiger is chasing you. Do you want to make slow, careful decisions or do you want to make quick decisions and trust your impulses? Fast decisions can keep us alive.

In the modern world, though, we rarely have to flee from a dangerous animal or search hard to find enough food. By all accounts, we are physically safe compared to our prehistoric ancestors. We should be able to *slow down*. Yet we spend our days running from goal to goal, never feeling like we have enough time, worrying about the mortgage, the next promotion and the opinions of others. We spend much of our time still seeming to fight or flee a predator.

PAUSE AND PLAN

Mindfulness is the antidote to the modern fight or flight syndrome. It enables us to shift into an alternative *pause and plan* mode, which involves slowing the heart rate, increasing sensitivity to the environment, and making cognitive processing more efficient. Mindfulness enables us to adjust our speed consciously—to slow down or speed up as the situation demands—and to respond with *intention* or *purpose*. Mindfulness gives us the mental space to ask the question, "What do I want to do in this moment?" or "What do I want to stand for now?" It helps us insert a mindful pause between our impulse to eat and the action of eating. Just one mindful breath can be all we need to gain control of our actions.

In the last two decades, there's been an explosion of research indicating the benefits of mindfulness practice. We now know that when we make mindfulness a habit, we can expect:

- better handling of negative events
- increased self-control
- better relationships with others
- reductions in chronic stress
- improved mental performance
- better ability to overcome bad habits.

This is why we call mindfulness the *ultimate habit*. Once we master it, the rest of our life is so much easier to manage.

What makes mindfulness difficult—and easy

Before we get started on making mindfulness a habit, we need to sound a warning: your mind will come up with a thousand reasons why you can't or don't have time to do it. Luckily, you already know what to do. When you hear your mind trying to talk you out of it, just let it chatter away like a radio playing in the background and stay with the mindfulness practice.

We all have plenty of time to practice mindfulness. We're awake for 16 hours or so each day, and we can use any of that time to practice mindfulness. We don't even have to do anything physically different from what we normally do. We could do exactly the same things we usually do, but just choose to do some of it mindfully. We could make our coffee mindfully, or eat breakfast mindfully, or interact with a friend mindfully. That's how easy it is to find the time.

The three hardest things about mindfulness practice will be:

1. Your mind will try hard to distract you; it will tell you all sorts of stories about how mindfulness practice is a waste of time or too difficult.
2. You'll feel like you want to stop the practice because some unpleasant emotion arises, such as boredom or frustration or anxiety.
3. Your mind will criticize you for not being good enough at mindfulness, or for not doing it right.

The great thing about mindfulness is that if any or all of those things do happen, you know you *are* doing it right. And—we know this will sound weird—if any or all of those things *don't* happen, you're also doing it right! Mindfulness isn't about *achieving* some excruciatingly difficult goal. It's about *noticing*: noticing what's happening here and now. You can notice whether you're bored or stimulated; you can notice whether your attention is wandering or not; you can notice whether your mind is chattering away or silent. And each time you notice, that's mindfulness!

In other words, it's impossible to do mindfulness practice incorrectly. The key is to notice when your attention wanders and gently bring it back, to notice the feeling of time pressure or distress and make space for it, to notice the self-criticism for not being good at mindfulness and thank your mind for turning even this practice of *simply noticing* into something to be judged. Mindfulness helps you stay with yourself—wandering attention, chattering mind, emotional discomfort and all.

Building the foundations for mindfulness

If a house has shoddy foundations, it will soon begin to sink. Cracks will appear in the walls and floors will warp. Similarly, if we don't have a firm foundation of mindfulness, we'll soon encounter problems with our other weight-loss habits. Without good mindfulness habits, we'll be quicker to fall into old, self-defeating patterns of behavior and slower to catch ourselves when our new, healthier habits are dropping off.

So, our primary aim is to establish a sturdy foundation of mindfulness upon which we can build our weight-loss habits. And the first step in building that foundation is to identify the three parts of the habit as outlined below (and illustrated in Figure 16):

1. WHAT IS THE *CUE* FOR MINDFULNESS PRACTICE?

We're much more likely to engage in regular practice if it's cued at a regular time. A cue might be a certain time of the day, such as when we wake up, or before our first cup of coffee, or immediately before lunch. The cue could also be a particular event or situation. Talking with another person can be a cue for mindful listening or walking your child to school can be a cue to be present for the duration of the walk. Sitting down for dinner may be a cue for mindful eating. Turning on the water in the shower may be a cue for mindful showering. Laying the kids" lunchboxes on the kitchen counter may be a cue for mindfully making packed lunches. Essentially, you want to commit to practicing something mindfully and be clear about the cue that will trigger that practice.

2. WHAT IS THE *ROUTINE* FOR MINDFULNESS PRACTICE?

What exactly does your mindfulness practice involve? Do you follow an ancient Eastern practice such as yoga, Tai Chi or sitting meditation? Or are you converting an everyday activity into a mindfulness practice? And either way, how do you start and end each session? (We'll give you some ideas for this below.)

3. WHAT IS THE *REWARD* FOR MINDFULNESS PRACTICE?

It's best if the reward is *intrinsic* to the routine. That means that when you do the mindfulness routine, it's fun, meaningful or useful to you. For example, mindfulness might help you to notice more about your physical environment, the taste and texture of your food, the emotional state of your friends, or to become more self-disciplined at your life goals. You might be quicker to catch a bad habit starting up and stop it in mid-flow; you may be quicker to notice cravings and allow them to flow through you without acting on them.

If you're struggling to notice what the intrinsic reward is, you can utilise an *extrinsic* reward. This is a reward that has nothing to do with mindfulness per se but is something you really want. For example, if you've succeeded at your mindfulness practice during the week, you can reward yourself at the end of the week with a movie or something else you love doing.

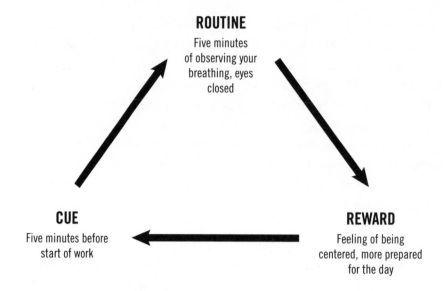

FIGURE 16: Example of a mindfulness routine

Finding a mindfulness routine that works for you

There's an infinite number of ways to practice mindfulness and there have been some exceptional books written on the topic. We find it best to help people experience mindfulness directly, rather than merely describing it in words, so we've included a few exercises in this chapter as possible examples of different kinds of mindfulness practice you can try. For more in-depth information on mindfulness, you could consult the list of recommended books at the end of this chapter.

It's important to be playful with mindfulness practices. Try out different ones. Give them time. If one activity doesn't work for you, try something else. Some people are great at doing sitting meditations while others dislike them intensely. If sitting still isn't your thing, you might try a walking or stretching meditation, or yoga, or developing mindfulness through everyday activities.

We understand how busy people are, and it's important to note that mindfulness practice can be very brief (less than five minutes) or a natural part of everyday living (i.e., you can practice mindfulness of an activity you're going to do anyway, so you don't need to find extra time to accommodate it). Mindfulness is a psychological skill, and as with all skills, the more practice you do, the better you get. And any practice, no matter how little, is better than none at all. If you do these activities for 10 minutes, that's obviously better than doing them for five minutes, but even if you only do them for one minute, that's better than not doing them at all. Every mindful moment makes a difference.

EXERCISE: SLOW BREATHING IN A FRANTIC WORLD

Deep, slow breathing is one of the best ways to activate the pause-and-plan system. Let's try this right now.

Place one hand on your chest and one on your abdomen. Now notice which hand is moving as you breathe. Most people notice that the chest hand moves. This is shallow breathing: the muscles of your ribcage are doing all the grunt work.

Deep breathing involves using your diaphragm, a huge sheet of muscle that separates your lungs from your abdomen. If your abdomen hand is moving rather than your chest hand, you're breathing deeply—that is to say, breathing from your diaphragm. As the diaphragm pulls the lungs fully open, it pushes the contents of the abdomen forwards. That's why you feel your abdomen hand moving, rather than your chest hand.

To learn how to breathe from your diaphragm, imagine you have a balloon in your stomach and you want to fill it. Inhale for three to six seconds until the "balloon" is filled, and then exhale for three to six seconds (the slower, the better) until it is completely empty. Do this for a minute, and notice how your body responds.

Almost everyone feels an instant sense of calm and peace as they breathe in this way. Very rarely, however, someone may actually feel light-headed or dizzy doing this. It is important for you to find a deep breathing level that is comfortable to you. There is no "right" way to do it. If the exercise causes you pain and discomfort, or if you have a medical condition (e.g., low blood pressure), you should stop it immediately and consult your doctor. Like everything in this book, you should experiment and see what works for you. Some people are comfortable with taking huge breaths, perhaps one every 16 seconds (8 seconds inhale, 8 seconds exhale), whereas others may prefer to breathe once every six seconds, or less. Still others may not want to take deep breaths, which is fine too. The key is to take slow breaths. Deep breathing helps with that, but is not the only way. You can also take slow normal breaths, just inhale and exhale slowly and pause for a couple of seconds in between.

It may seem unbelievable that something as simple as breathing could be so crucial to your weight-loss goals, but breathing is the first way of building and practicing the essential skill of mindfulness, which is the foundation of all the other skills and habits that will help you lose weight effectively.

EXERCISE: COUNTING THE BREATH

This variation on the breathing exercise involves counting each exhalation until you get to 10 and then starting again. It does not require you to engage in deep breathing. Any breath is just right (though you can choose to deep breathe if you wish).

With your first breath in the sequence, breathe in and, as you breathe out, silently say to yourself, "One." As you exhale your next breath, silently say to yourself, "Two." And so on. Once you've reached 10, go back to one. If at any time you lose count, simply go back to one and start again.

Like deep breathing, counting the breath will tend to activate your pause and plan system. You can expect your mind to distract you, repeatedly. Notice when this happens, then gently bring your attention back to your breath. Sometimes you'll have trouble getting past three before you get lost. That is perfectly natural.

Instead of counting, you could use a mantra. Mantra meditation is often done with the eyes closed and involves silently chanting a single word or phrase. If you wish to do this, pick a phrase that has personal meaning for you. You might, for example, repeat "kindness" or "calming" over and over again. Or you might repeat a phrase such as "I am present now."

The point of this exercise is not for the words to have some hypnotic power over you. Mantra meditation doesn't require you to be religious or believe in anything mystical. In fact, if you repeat any word for more than a minute, it will often lose all meaning and become just a rhythmic sound. Mantra meditation gives you something clear to focus on, and tends to disrupt rumination and worrying. If you use the same mantra each time, you may discover that you can also use it in the flow of everyday life, especially during stressful times. The mantra will then help you slow down and make effective decisions.

EXERCISE: THE MINDFUL JUMPSTART

Although we suggest 10 minutes here, this exercise can be done for a very short time, say as little as three minutes just before a difficult meeting, or for longer periods. We call it a jumpstart because it can be a way to refresh yourself for the day and help you to focus on what you care about. It consists of three steps:

1. You notice your breathing and other experiences in your body for about a minute.
2. You repeat a simple phrase, such as "I'm present now."
3. After about 10 minutes, you finish and state your intention for the day: "Today I will . . ." (e.g., be mindful, kind, courageous, etc.)

Be careful not to turn the mindful jumpstart into some torturous activity that must be done exactly right. Don't think of mindfulness activities as yet another thing you must do, but rather as something you choose to do for yourself. There's no better way to refresh and refocus yourself on the things that are important to you in life.

Close your eyes and begin with about a minute of just being aware of your breath. Simply notice your breath—there's no need to shorten or lengthen it or do anything else to it. Just let it be and notice that breathing, like so much in our life, occurs without any effort. If you get distracted by other sensations in your body, that's fine. Notice that, then gently bring yourself back to your breath. Sometimes a worrying thought will intrude. That's perfectly fine too. Just notice it and let it go. Don't cling to it. If it wants to stick around, don't push it away. Just let your thoughts and feelings be, and gently bring yourself back to your breath.

After about a minute of noticing your breath, start repeating, "I'm present now." If you practice the phrase when you're sitting peacefully like this, it means that later, when you're facing a stressful situation, you can repeat the phrase to yourself and it will help you become mindful and present, and reduce your stress. Keep repeating this phrase for nine minutes, if you have time; we recommend using an alarm of some sort to signal when the total 10 minutes are up, so you don't have to keep looking at a clock. (Try to choose a calming sound for your alarm, such as a chime, rather than something raucous like a klaxon; mobile phone apps are perfect for this.)

Once the alarm sounds, do one last thing: silently state your intention for the day, beginning with the words, "Today I will . . ." and completing the sentence. Think about the quality you want to impart to your actions throughout the day. For example, you might say, "Today I will be fully present to my partner" or "Today I will choose a healthy option for lunch" or "Today I will stay focused on the task that's important to me" or "Today I will treat each person I meet with kindness."

EXERCISE: **EVERYDAY MINDFULNESS**

Every moment in your life offers an opportunity to practice mindfulness. You can be mindful during a walk, talking to others, playing with your children, listening to music, showering, drinking coffee, washing the dishes, sweeping the floor, and so on. We recommend you practice being mindful of at least one activity per day. Try this for a week and see how your perceptions change over that time.

As you are doing the activity, pay careful attention to your sensations. If you're showering, what does it feel like? What thoughts are popping into your head? Notice your movements as you wash or bend. If you're brushing your teeth, notice the taste of the toothpaste, the sensation on your gums, and so on.

We are so often caught up in our heads that we don't notice the people around us. Sometimes we don't even notice or hear our loved ones. Mindfulness of others involves paying full attention to what they are saying and seeking to connect as much as possible with their experience in the moment. Being present to another is often the greatest gift we can give them. Try it as many times as you can today.

Joseph: the space between two goals

I would like to share one of my experiences in increasing the extent I engage in mindful physical activity. I am always in a rush and don't feel like I have time to do anything except complete the goals of the day. Sometimes I feel like I am in a high-pressure race, running around and around a track. I wonder what it would be like to step off the track and just sit down in the stands. Could I just sit there?

I decided to commit to an activity designed to give me a break from the race and decrease my sedentary behavior. Instead of driving my seven-year-old daughter to school, I would walk her to school and delay work by 30 minutes. I found this goal surprisingly hard. I experienced tension and the recurring thought "You don't have time for this."

Thank goodness I made space for these feelings and thoughts and committed to my activity. The walk to school has become one of the most meaningful moments of my day. Sometimes my daughter, Grace, is present to the outside world, picking flowers and noticing interesting trees and animals. I stay with her mindfully, and she helps pull me into the physical world. Sometimes she is not present, worrying about a bully in school or her math class. I am present to her then too, and she talks to me about these things. Sometimes she talks to me about singing in front of a large crowd like Katy Perry. I am present to all of it and I am pulled out of my self-absorbed world into a world that we experience together. In these in-between moments I feel fully connected and alive.

Mindful eating

Have you ever felt overfull, perhaps even bloated or in pain, after eating too much? Do you sometimes eat snacks while working, and don't even notice until the snack is all gone? Do you ever munch your way through a huge box of popcorn or a bag of candy at the movies, or snack thoughtlessly on whatever is available in the kitchen? Do you tend to overeat automatically when you're at a party or socializing? These are all examples of *mindless eating*. Most mindless eating is *not* driven by genuine hunger or the biological needs of our body. Rather, it's driven by cues in the environment such as fast-food ads. Non-hungry eating is a major cause of weight gain. Mindful eating is the cure.

Mindful eating involves paying deliberate, curious attention to the experience of eating. You practice noticing everything about your food: the shape, color, taste, texture and smell, and even the movements of your teeth and jaws and the sounds you make when you chew and swallow. Mindful eating also involves paying attention to your internal body cues, such as those that indicate your level of hunger.

When you eat mindfully, you'll not only intensify your enjoyment of your food, you'll be satisfied with smaller amounts of it. You'll notice which foods you really love and which you don't like so much, which foods make you feel healthy or energized and which make you feel sluggish or unhealthy. You might then choose to eat different types or amounts of food. You might eat chocolate mindfully, for example, and discover you really don't like the taste of a certain brand. You might, therefore, decide to switch brands.

HOW TO EAT MINDFULLY

Mindful eating helps you connect better with what you love and helps you decide how much you eat based on your own core values (see Chapter 1). Here are some tips to make your eating more mindful:

1. Slow down the pace of eating.
2. Eat away from distractions, such as television.
3. Observe your body's hunger and fullness cues, and use these to guide when you begin and end eating.
4. Eat food that's both pleasing and nourishing, and use all your senses while you eat it.
5. Get fully involved in your food. Be curious about the varieties of vegetables, fruit, legumes, and so on.
6. Be experimental! Eat silently with the family, if possible. Or eat the first part of your meal mindfully. Even one minute of mindfulness can change your eating behavior for the better.

Create a personalized mindfulness plan

It's all too easy to forget to engage in mindfulness practice, just as it's easy to slip off a diet. The best way to remember is to make mindfulness part of your routine. We therefore encourage you to generate a mindfulness plan along the lines of the example from our author Joseph in the table opposite. It is important to note that Joseph doesn't do all these exercises every day, and there are some days he doesn't do any of them. The important thing is to keep doing your best and returning to your practice, no matter how many times you forget or skip it.

Start by taking some time to think about what mindfulness routines you'd like to engage in. Then describe the regular cue, routine and reward for each of these. It's a good idea to put your plan somewhere prominent so you'll remember to do it. You might also want to leave yourself reminder notes or put a reminder in your phone. Mindfulness practice isn't hard in and of itself; the hardest thing about it is remembering to do it! Remember also that even small steps can start tipping us toward a better life (Chapter 3). If you can't commit to lots of mindfulness routines, just commit to one small one. Start with that and see what happens.

JOSEPH'S MINDFULNESS PLAN

CUE (WHAT AND WHEN)	ROUTINE	REWARD
Making a cup of coffee first thing in the morning	• 10 seconds of mindful breathing with empty cup in hand • Notice each step of the coffee-making process • Notice when distracted, bring self back	• Strengthened attention • Reminded of the value of mindfulness
Just before I start work	• Mindful observation of breath	• Day more focused on values • Decreased stress • Lowered reactivity to unimportant events
Walking to school with my daughter	• During walk, attend to my daughter and notice all that's around me • When I notice myself becoming absorbed by my mind, gently return my attention to the outside world and to my daughter	• Greater connection with daughter • Greater receptivity to outside experiences
Eating breakfast	• For the first minute eat my breakfast mindfully	• Greater enjoyment of food • Improved decision-making around food

MINDFULNESS RESOURCES

Mindfulness: A Practical Guide to Finding Peace in a Frantic World by Mark Williams & Daniel Penmen (Piatkus, London, 2011).

This excellent book will take you through a wide variety of meditations and show you how to insert mindfulness into your everyday life. The hard copy of the book includes a CD and the ebook version incorporates audio. This is a good starting point to develop your mindfulness practice.

After the Ecstasy, the Laundry: How the Heart Grows Wise on the Spiritual Path by Jack Kornfield (Bantam, New York, 2000).

This book does an excellent job of connecting mindfulness to spiritual growth, and is well worth reading for those interested in this area. The book illustrates how mindfulness can lead to wisdom, deep compassion and freedom, but also does not ignore the ordinary moments of doing the laundry, and experiencing sadness, anxiety, confusion, and struggle.

Unlearning Meditation: What to Do When the Instructions Get in the Way by Jason Siff (Shambhala Publications, Boston, Massachusetts, 2010).

This practical book does an excellent job of helping people who struggle with meditation and meditation "rules." Of course most of the rules are probably coming from our own desire to create rules and turn meditation practice into another thing to "achieve." This book will give you plenty of advice and alternatives for meditation practice.

SUMMARY: IF YOU WISH TO LOSE WEIGHT . . .

DO MORE OF THIS	DO LESS OF THIS
Make mindfulness a routine. It will be the core skill to help you break old habits and build new ones.	Practice mindfulness haphazardly. Don't bother to establish a routine and just hope you'll remember to practice.
Remember that loss of concentration, getting distracted by thoughts and wandering attention are all recurring aspects of mindfulness practice. There is no right or wrong way to practice mindfulness.	Believe there's only one right way to practice mindfulness and turn it into another thing to beat yourself up about. Hold tightly to the idea that the only way to learn mindfulness is by sitting on a cushion meditating. Fail to notice that every life moment offers a chance to practice mindfulness.
Practice mindful eating regularly.	Eat rapidly and without noticing.
Be creative. Eating a meal mindfully for even one minute—or even one mouthful—can make a difference.	Hold tightly to the belief that you never have time for mindful eating.

8.
MAKING HARD CHOICES EASIER

If we are to lose weight and keep it off, we are going to have to make many hard choices. Sometimes we will find ourselves in the middle of a craving wave and feel like we simply *must* eat a treat, or we will feel stressed out and tempted to visit the nearest fast-food chain. The more of these tough choices we have in the day, the more likely we are to give in. We can use the skills in this book to help us with these tough decisions, but wouldn't it be great if we could make life a little easier? Wouldn't it be great if we could reduce temptation and make the healthy choice easy and automatic? The good news is, we can. This chapter will show you how.

Weight gain is rarely if ever due to one single behavior. Usually it's the result of a number of small, bad habits, such as always having something sweet after dinner, or regularly stopping at a fast-food restaurant after a stressful day at work. We learned from the previous chapter that all habits follow the same pattern: there's a cue from the environment (e.g., you see jelly beans on the table) or internally (e.g., a feeling of boredom or anxiety), there's a routine (e.g., you grab a few jelly beans and mindlessly eat them), and then there's a reward (e.g., a sweet taste and a sugar rush).

To break any bad habit you need to change one of the three components of the habit loop: you need to eliminate or modify the cue, alter the routine or change the reward. This chapter will show you how to change the first part of the habit loop—the cue. Through this we'll show you just how powerful cues are, how they exist all around us and how, with a few simple changes to your environment, you can reduce or even eliminate many of your bad eating habits.

Figure 17 below illustrates how a simple change in cues can alter the eating routine.

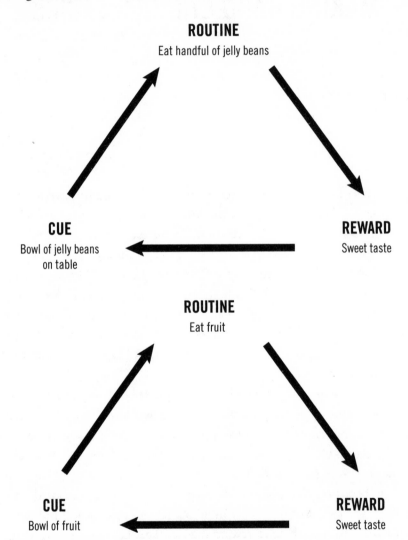

FIGURE 17: Altering the cue in the habit loop. The bad habit of the first loop can be turned into a good habit simply by changing the cue.

THE EATING CUES WE NEVER NOTICE

The greatest trick the devil ever played was convincing the world that he did not exist.

—Charles Baudelaire

Do you know how habits develop? Or why you make the choices you make? Or how much of your eating behavior is a conscious choice rather than an automatic reaction to cues in the environment? Most of us believe we're fully aware of what influences us. Most of us are wrong.

We're often unaware of all the cues in the environment telling us what to eat and how much to eat. Think about something as simple as going to the supermarket. The moment we enter the door, we're bombarded with advertising. Packages have phrases like "all natural," "healthy," "authentic French," "satisfy your appetite," "indulgent," "world-famous," and "original." Much of the advertising is subtle and indirect. The packages are illustrated with images of smiling children, beautiful women picking flowers in the sunshine, "healthy" checkmarks, and images of medals and ribbons. Marketing experts have designed each of these images with the sole purpose of influencing you.

And so far we've just been talking about our time in the supermarket. What about the rest of our lives? We're bombarded with cues to eat and drink when we travel to work, listen to the radio, read a magazine, go to the movies, surf the net or watch TV.

It's difficult for us to admit we're actually influenced by these ads. We know someone is influenced by them, but surely it's not *us*! The problem is, the more we're in denial or ignorant of those unconscious influences on our behavior, the greater their impact on us.

Seven surprising sources of influence

Here are seven scientific findings that show just how unaware we are of what influences us:

1. We'll tend to eat a much larger serving if a food is labeled "low-fat" than if it doesn't have this label.

2. We'll tend to believe that a food tastes better if it has an attractive name. For example, we'd probably prefer the taste of caviar, kiwifruit and escargots over the flavor of fish eggs, Chinese gooseberries and snails, even though they're exactly the same foods.

3. We tend to eat more old, stale popcorn from a big container than fresh popcorn from a small container. The size of the container influences how much we eat.

4. We'll eat 69 percent more jelly beans when all the colors are mixed together than if they're separated into individual colors. The variety of food influences how much we eat.

5. The more people we have dinner with, the more we'll eat. We'll eat more food with two friends than with one. We'll eat even more food with three friends than with two.

6. If our eating companions eat a lot of food, we'll also tend to eat a lot of food.

7. If we have a large meal, we'll tend to underestimate how many calories we've eaten. If, for example, we think we've just eaten 1,000 calories, we've probably eaten closer to 1,400 calories!

Making decisions about food

Every time we make a food decision, we're subject to unconscious influences. How many such decisions do you think you make in a day? What will you eat for breakfast? How much will you eat? Will you have that dessert after dinner? Will you have that snack in front of the TV or in the car or while you're reading the paper? Will you go out or stay in or get takeaway? What will you cook tonight? And so on, and so on. Before you read on to the next paragraph take a wild guess at the answer to this question: how many food-related decisions do you think you make in a day?

Believe it or not, research suggests that we make *more than 200* food decisions a day, or approximately 6,000 per month. If you underestimated, you're not alone. Most people are unaware of how many food decisions they make. Most people are also unaware of what causes them to eat. We think we're making decisions based on hunger and desire, but really our eating is influenced by such superficial things as the size of a bowl, the shape of a drinking glass and the number of people we're eating with.

Earlier in the book, we showed you how to make mindful food choices that fit with the values you identified in Chapter 1. But can we really make 200 mindful choices a day? Does *anyone* have that much energy? It's not likely, is it? Realistically, we're still going to make many choices mindlessly.

The good news is, these "mindless choices" don't have to work against us. What if we could modify our environment so that our mindless choices were consistent with our health and diet goals? What if we could deliberately redesign our environment so it "tells" us to eat less?

Redesigning your environment so you eat less

Here are six tips for redesigning your environment to alter your eating cues and reduce your food intake.

1. "MINI-SIZE ME"

Someone puts a beautiful bowl of soup in front of you. How much of it would you eat? When would you stop eating it? Most people say, "I'd stop eating when I'm full." That's a reasonable belief, but it turns out to be completely wrong.

Brian Wansink, a scientist at Cornell University, decided to investigate what causes people to stop eating a meal. He and his colleagues gave people bowls of soup and allowed them to eat as much as they wanted for 20 minutes. What the people eating the soup *didn't* know was that some of the soup bowls were continuously being refilled by a hidden tube. In other words, they were bottomless bowls that would never run out of soup. The other bowls in this study were completely normal.

The people with the bottomless bowls ate *73 percent more* soup than the people with the normal bowls. And perhaps even more surprising, the people with the bottomless bowls *didn't realize* they'd eaten so much more.

The moral of the story is, most of us *don't* use our sense of hunger or fullness to tell us when to stop eating. Rather, if we see food, we eat it. Many of us will eat everything on our plate, and the larger the plate the more food we'll eat.

And right there is a big part of the problem, because since the 1970s, portion sizes have increased in restaurants, in supermarkets and at home. The classic cookbook *The Joy of Cooking* has constantly been revised over the years since its first publication in 1931, and the serving sizes have become steadily larger. In 1936, the average recipe to serve four people had about 2,100 calories. By 2006, the average recipe had exploded to 3,051 calories!

In a more humorous approach, Brian Wansink and his colleagues also analysed 52 of the best known depictions of the Last Supper over the 1000 years from 1000 c.e. They assessed the size of loaves of bread, main dishes and plates (relative to the head sizes of the people in the painting). The size of the main course increased by a whopping 69.2 percent, bread by 23.1 percent and the plate size by 65.6 percent. Clearly, our cultural notion of a "normal" amount of food has increased, along with the size of our waist.

If we're driven to eat more when we see more, we can also re-engineer our environment so that we see less and eat less. Here are four practical suggestions from Brian Wansink for things you can do straight away to redesign your environment.

- **Use small containers.** People tend to eat what they see in front of them rather than stop eating when they've had enough. If you buy food in large containers, you'll probably eat more of it, so put smaller portions into smaller containers (snap-lock bags or air-tight containers).
- **Work by the "half-plate rule."** One half of your plate should be filled with vegetables and fruit, the other with protein (e.g., meat) and/or carbohydrates (e.g., pasta, potato, bread, rice).
- **Put your whole meal on your plate.** Put everything you want to eat on a plate before you start eating it. If you have a whole lot of serving dishes on the table in front of you, you're far more likely to help yourself to extra servings.
- **Use smaller plates and bowls to serve your food.** It's quite amazing how effective this is for most people. A serving of food that looks tiny on a gigantic plate looks far more substantial

when you serve it in a small bowl, so even though you're eating the same amount, psychologically you may find it far more satisfying.

These four visual tricks will help remind you to eat modest portion sizes that satisfy your hunger. There's some danger, however, that we can be "too reassured" by these tricks and become mindless about how much we're eating. Just because you're eating off a small dinner plate, doesn't mean you no longer have to think about how much you're eating. You might actually end up eating as much food as you would have using a larger plate, especially if you pile your food up high on the small plate or go back for seconds and thirds. So use these four suggestions mindfully.

2. INCREASE THE VARIETY OF HEALTHY FOODS

Research suggests the greater the variety of foods in front of us, the more we'll eat because we tend to grow tired of eating the same thing. The dark side of this variety effect is that if we're offered a wide variety of fatty foods (e.g., cake and ice cream), we'll tend to eat more than if we're offered a single fatty food. The bright side of the variety effect is that if we're offered a wide variety of fruit and vegetables, we will probably eat more of these.

So the trick here is to decrease the variety of unhealthy foods you eat and increase the variety of healthy foods. If, for example, you're at a buffet or party with lots of tempting, high-calorie food, make a commitment to eat only one or two unhealthy varieties.

To increase the variety of healthy foods you can be playful: try fruit, vegetables and legumes that are new to you, and find new ways of combining them to produce delicious meals. You might try having two or three different vegetables at dinnertime, for example. We think you'll find it easier to eat five bites of two different vegetables than 10 bites of the same vegetable.

3. REDUCE DISTRACTIONS WHEN YOU'RE EATING

Research shows that we eat more when watching a TV show or movie, listening to the radio, working on the computer or reading the paper.

This means that if you want to cut down on mindless eating, one of the best things you can do is eat when you're not distracted (or not eat when you are).

You don't have to make major changes in your life to reduce distracted eating. Look for little opportunities: could you switch off the TV or radio, or put down the book or newspaper, or set the computer or iPhone aside? Many people find this incredibly difficult, so it's often useful to start small: aim to eat mindfully for the first minute of your meal. Once you can do that, aim to eat mindfully for the first two minutes. If you can eat mindfully for five minutes, you're doing incredibly well. Can you commit to this one small step right now?

4. EAT MINDFULLY WITH OTHER PEOPLE

As we noted above, the more people you eat with, the more you eat. People tend to eat 28 percent more food with one person than on their own, 53 percent more with three people, and a whopping 76 percent more with six people. In concrete terms, a 76 percent increase will make a 250-gram steak balloon to 450 grams and will turn 30 fries into more than 50 fries. You can bet those extra calories will expand your waistline!

Food and our social life are so intertwined that it would be impossible to split them. We want to hang out with our friends and family and eat good food as we do. The good news is that we can still do that while maintaining our diet goals. The key is to eat with intention and mindfully. Think about how much you want to eat before you eat (intention). If, for example, you're going to an Indian restaurant with a group of friends, you might decide beforehand to have only one samosa, two-thirds of a serving of butter chicken, half a serving of plain rice and half a garlic naan. You could also slow down your pace of eating and drink more water. Savor your food and enjoy your time with friends and family.

5. SEE LESS, EAT LESS

A wealth of research shows that if we see food, we tend to eat it. People eat more chocolate, for example, if it's easily within reach and they can see it sitting in a clear bowl. Similarly, people tend to eat more sandwiches if they're wrapped in see-through wrapping rather than opaque wrapping. Other research suggests that buying in bulk or stockpiling food can lead to greater food consumption.

Simple changes to your environment can reduce the amount you eat mindlessly. Don't put treats in the middle of the dining room table; put them away in a cupboard and put a bowl of fruit on the table instead. Similarly, put your chocolate biscuits in a tin, close the lid, and place it on the highest shelf of the pantry. Don't stockpile unhealthy food.

6. PLAN IN ORDER TO AVOID THE "DESPERATE ZONE"

It's very hard to make workable decisions about food when we're extremely hungry or have entered the *desperate zone*. We know we're in the desperate zone when we're ravenous: we're craving food and feel like we have to eat something right away. Once we're in this state, we're highly likely to go for convenience foods that are instantly available to eat. Alas, many convenience foods are high-fat or high-sugar junk foods.

To avoid this trap, we need to plan ahead. Take a moment to think about when you're most likely to be in the desperate zone. Is it straight after work or perhaps at breakfast tea? When you go on a day outing without a packed lunch? The key is to anticipate and plan. Know when you typically enter the desperate zone and have a snack readily available, ideally a healthy one. Muffins and muesli bars are loaded to the brim with sugar and fat, so they're not a great choice if you want to lose weight. Bananas, apples, grapes, carrots and celery, on the other hand, are incredibly healthy convenience foods. (So are nuts, but they're loaded with calories, so keep your portions small.)

SUMMARY: IF YOU WISH TO LOSE WEIGHT . . .

DO MORE OF THIS	DO LESS OF THIS
Recognize that you're often unaware of the factors that cause you to eat.	Insist that you're aware of all the things that make you eat.
Be curious about your eating patterns and notice times when you eat more than you intended (e.g., when you're with other people, when you're distracted, when you're in the desperate zone described above).	Fail to notice the times and places when you eat more calories than you intended.
Redesign your environment so you're likely to eat less.	Ignore factors in the environment that lead you to eat more.

9.
FINDING LASTING MOTIVATION

We offer you one promise throughout this book: *we'll tell you the truth*. We'll guide you based on the best available scientific evidence. We believe the truth has one major advantage: it gives you the best chance of enjoying a full, healthy and meaningful life. We turn now to a particularly difficult truth.

Motivation doesn't last

Have you ever gone on a diet and succeeded for a short time? Perhaps you lost weight and started feeling good about yourself. Everything seemed to be going well. Then one day you stopped losing weight. You plateaued. You couldn't seem to take any more weight off, no matter how little you ate, no matter how hungry you let yourself feel.

And then it happened: the return. Ever so slowly, the weight crept back on, pound upon pound, until you were back to your original weight, or—shock horror!—even heavier than before.

And there's something even worse than gaining the weight. It's what our judgmental mind does to us next. Our mind will say we've failed at another diet. It will accuse us of being undisciplined and weak. Maybe our mind will start comparing us with other, thinner people, and we'll feel angry with ourselves or depressed or hopeless. "They" seem to be able to eat whatever they want and not gain any weight. "So what's wrong with you?" says our mind. Sometimes we want to shout out, "This is unfair!" And we'd be right. It *is* unfair.

We're not built for losing weight. Our bodies are designed to store fat, not lose it. Remember, many thousands of years ago, humans lived in environments where there was often not enough food. Those humans needed to be good at storing calories (i.e., fat) in their body when food was available, and at conserving calories when food was scarce. Naturally, those who were best at conserving calories were more likely to survive periods of food scarcity.

To illustrate this point, imagine two cavewomen, Lucy and Cynthia. When there's plenty of food, Lucy gains weight like crazy. In contrast, Cynthia doesn't gain weight. If Lucy had a modern mind, she might look at her sister and feel a bit jealous. "How come *she* gets to eat anything and not gain weight?" But what happens when a hard winter hits? Or when there's a famine? Who's more likely to survive? Not slim Cynthia: she has no fat in reserve. Lucy is the one who survives.

The survivors, like Lucy, were our ancestors, and we carry their fat-conserving genetic code.

Now fast-forward to the present day. High-calorie food is plentiful, we don't experience famines, and because our lifestyle is so much less physically active than that of our ancestors, we burn up much less energy than they did.

Yet our body hasn't changed. It's still genetically programmed to store energy in the form of fat. So if we go on a diet and start reducing calories, our body naturally goes into conservation mode—just as it would have done thousands of years ago during a famine—and actively resists our attempts to keep the weight off.

This fight occurs via a number of interrelated biological systems that influence our metabolism (i.e., how much energy we burn), our hunger, and our preference for fat and sugar. The metabolism of people who've lost weight through dieting is significantly slower than the metabolism of other people of exactly the same weight who *did not* diet. Indeed, a formerly overweight person must eat about 350 calories per day *less* to maintain the same body weight as someone similar who's never been overweight. And if that isn't bad enough, people who've lost weight are more likely to be hungrier than those who *haven't* lost weight, and they also prefer food high in sugar and fat.

Now let's say we overcome all these biological biases and keep the weight off for a year. Does our body go back to normal? The bad news is no. Our body still fights to regain the weight even years after we lost it.

That *is* unfair! But it's also liberating. Why? Because it means our struggle to keep the weight off is *natural*. It's not a sign of weakness. It's part of the body's design to do whatever it can to regain lost weight. There are no exceptions. When we lose weight, our body follows its DNA programming to conserve calories and actively seek out foods rich in sugar and fat. We're not to blame for this!

We *can* lose weight

There is hope. Even though we're blameless when it comes to our past struggles, we can still act to improve our future. Sustained weight loss *is* possible. Here are some statistics to illustrate the point:

- Sixty-two percent of people who were once overweight have, at some point, managed to lose at least 10 percent of their maximum weight.
- Among those who lost at least 10 percent of their maximum weight, 47–49 percent maintained that loss for at least one year and 25–27 percent maintained it for five years or longer.

So weight loss is *not* easy, but it *is* possible. And it certainly gets easier when we know what we're up against in setting out to lose that weight. We know our biology is going to make it hard to keep the weight off. We know we're going to experience setbacks. And we know that when we fail:

1. Our mind will criticize us and turn us into a problem to be solved (see Chapter 4).
2. We won't want the emotional distress of failure and will seek desperately to push it away (see Chapter 2).
3. We may try to push away the distress either by going to the extreme of fad diets or by rejecting all diets and making up reasons why we can't succeed at weight loss (see Chapter 5).

In summary, we know we'll struggle to lose weight and we know our mind will beat us up when we fail. So how can we stay motivated when we experience setbacks?

Reacting to failure

Here's what John (see John's story in Chapter 4) thinks: "I need to be hard on myself to stay motivated. If I don't feel like exercising, I kick myself in the ass by saying things like, 'Come on, get off your fat ass and do something.' I sometimes hate myself for being so lazy."

Let's take a closer look at John's inner critic. Imagine this critic was actually outside his body and you could overhear it talking. You walk by while it's saying to John, "Come on, get off your fat ass and do something." How would you react?

Does your mind ever speak to you in a similar manner to John's? When you fail to live up to your ideals, does your inner critic say mean things to you? If your mind does this, you're not alone. We're all capable of anger, blame and harsh judgment. We readily direct it to the outside world and we easily turn it inwards, upon ourselves. Here's a quick quiz to help you become more aware of your own inner critic.

ONE-MINUTE QUIZ: **HOW HARD ARE YOU ON YOURSELF?**

Do you beat yourself up when you make mistakes? Do you think you have to be perfect? Or do you give yourself a break now and then?

SELF-CRITICISM	HOW OFTEN DO YOU LISTEN TO THIS SELF-CRITICISM?				
	NEVER	RARELY	SOMETIMES	OFTEN	ALWAYS
I'm intolerant of the parts of myself I don't like.	0	1	2	3	4
In hard times, I don't take care of myself.	0	1	2	3	4
I feel disgusted with my body.	0	1	2	3	4
I hate myself when I lose self-control.	0	1	2	3	4
I beat myself up if I don't exercise as much as I intended to.	0	1	2	3	4
I feel ashamed when I overeat.	0	1	2	3	4
I feel worthless.	0	1	2	3	4

How many items did you rate as 2 or 3 or even higher? If you rated many items as 3 or more (i.e., you scored between 24 and 32), this may indicate that your critical mind can be quite busy, especially during difficult times.

We've already learned how to defuse from self-critical thoughts (see Chapter 4) so they don't dominate us, but this raises an important question: do we *need* self-criticism in order to stay motivated? Can we motivate ourselves with kindness instead? Or are we afraid of being kind to ourselves? Try this one-minute quiz to see.

ONE-MINUTE QUIZ: **ARE YOU AFRAID OF BEING KIND TO YOURSELF?**

Do you think you have to suffer in order to be a better person? Do you think you can't reward yourself until your life is perfect?

UNKIND STATEMENT	HOW OFTEN DO YOU FUSE WITH THIS STATEMENT?				
	NEVER	RARELY	SOMETIMES	OFTEN	ALWAYS
If I'm kind to myself, I'll become weak.	0	1	2	3	4
If I don't criticize myself, my flaws will show and everybody will see them.	0	1	2	3	4
If I'm kind to myself, my standards will drop.	0	1	2	3	4
If I'm kind to myself, I'll become overwhelmed by sadness.	0	1	2	3	4
If I don't criticize myself, others will reject me.	0	1	2	3	4
If I accept my flaws, bad things will happen.	0	1	2	3	4
I don't deserve kindness.	0	1	2	3	4
If I'm kind to myself, I'll start eating unhealthy foods.	0	1	2	3	4
If I'm kind to myself, I'll lose control.	0	1	2	3	4

How many items did you rate as 2 or 3 or even higher? If you rated many items as 3 or more (i.e., you scored between 27 and 36), this suggests that you're afraid of being kind to yourself. So let's explore kindness and see if it really does make you weak.

Abuse is not inspiring

Imagine you work for an abusive boss who for the sake of our example happens to be a man. He talks to you in an angry voice and says things like, "You're not doing enough. You're lazy and good for nothing." He tells you you're disgusting and stupid and that he hates you. Even when you do something well, he doesn't compliment you. He only shakes his head and says you could have done better.

If you actually worked for a bully like this, how motivated would you be to perform well? Would you feel inspired to get up early in the morning and work hard? Or would you become stressed, drained, resentful and unmotivated? Would you maybe even rebel against him, deliberately doing a bad job and ignoring what he says?

Research shows very clearly that self-criticism (letting the abusive boss dominate) doesn't lead to better outcomes. Rather, it leads to:

- lower motivation to exercise and higher likelihood of giving up
- lower wellbeing
- worse response to negative life events
- worse response to failure, and lower motivation to improve oneself.

But you don't even have to look at the research. Just check out your own experience. When you have a setback or a failure and you start beating yourself up about it, what's the typical outcome? Does berating yourself actually improve your situation? Does it make you a better person in the long run? Does it make you feel more inspired and motivated, or less?

When you can no longer rely on your inner critic for motivation, what then is your alternative?

Being kind to yourself

We're so used to being hard on ourselves that we actually have to learn how to treat ourselves kindly. Isn't that crazy? You don't have to teach cats how to be kind to themselves. They'll treat themselves nicely and eat a tasty meal whenever it's available. They'll sleep whenever and wherever they feel like it. Unlike us, they won't attack themselves in order to get motivated. In contrast, most of us are so used to self-punishment that it feels almost unnatural to be kind to ourselves. The figure on page 165 illustrates how we find our way to self-kindness, and we will now do some exercises that will help us put kindness into action.

EXERCISE: FINDING A KIND FRIEND INSIDE YOURSELF

A good way to start is by thinking about people who've been kind and encouraging to you in the past. Really see if you can pull up the details and emotions from that memory. How did the kind person behave? What qualities of action did they put into play; for example, were they forgiving, supportive, helpful, gentle, encouraging, nurturing, providing, empathetic, kind, trusting, accepting?

These are "kind values." They're ways we could choose to act toward another person, perhaps someone we love or care about. They're also ways we could choose to act toward ourselves. Here are three simple steps you can use to create kindness in your life.

1. **Notice and name your inner critic**
   We assume you've already been practicing this (see Chapter 4), but if not, it's never too late to start. Let's try it now.
   Notice: Think about a time when you were struggling and really beating yourself up. Try to bring that memory into the present moment and relive the emotions. Listen for your inner critic. What were you saying to yourself in that memory?
   Notice: What does your inner critic sound like in the memory? Is it angry, self-righteous or defeated? Is it soft or loud? Is it talking fast or slow?
   Notice: What was your inner voice criticizing you for? Your appearance, career, self-control, relationships? Is this typical?
   Name: If you could give your inner critic a name, what would it be? It might be: The Judge, Miss Angry, the Slasher, the Grim Reaper, the Abuser, the Dominator, the Assassin, the Inner Bastard, the Inner Bitch, the Inquisitor. Come up with your own name now. (If you can't think of one, it's okay to stick with "the inner critic" or use one of our examples.)

2. **Defuse and make space for your inner critic**
   Instead of fighting your inner critic, acknowledge its presence, using the name you just gave it. So, if you called your critic the Dominator, you might say,

"Hello, Dominator" or "There goes the Dominator again" or "Thanks for shar-ing, Dominator." This step will help you step back, or *defuse*, from the critic.

Notice that this inner critic doesn't have to interfere with what you care about. The angry critic can make its angry noise, and we can still do what's important to us. Our inner critic can't stop us heading in the direction we want to go.

3. **Be a kind friend to yourself**

How does your mind treat you when you don't live up to its expectations? Does it turn you into a problem to be solved? Now that you've noticed, named and made room for this inner critic that wants to solve you, let's shift gears and practice kindness.

Can you speak to yourself the way a kind friend would speak to you? Imagine this friend knows everything about you, even your "worst flaws." Yet this friend still likes you and accepts you. The friend wants you to be successful and take care of yourself when you fail.

YOUR KIND FRIEND IN ACTION

Here's what your kind friend might say to you, following the steps above, when you've failed to live up to a health goal (you went off the diet, say, or you gained a couple of pounds).

1. "Wow, you're having a rough day, [your name]. Your inner critic is coming down hard on you. You didn't act like you wanted to, and now you're beating yourself up."

2. "That's okay. Those feelings are natural. Everyone has them. You can make space for them and they'll come and go. There's no need to fight them."

3. "You know, everybody fails at their goals sometimes. You can still be kind to yourself. What can you do, my good friend, to give yourself the self-care you need during this hard time? Take a long bath? Talk to a friend? Or just take some time out to see a movie? It takes courage to recommit to goals when you fail. Would you be willing to do that now? Would you be able to gently encourage yourself to recommit to your health goals?"

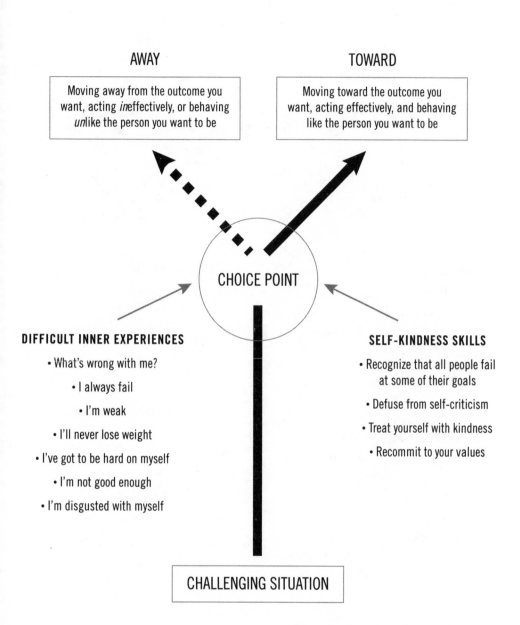

FIGURE 18: Practice self-kindness and stop punishing yourself

SUMMARY: IF YOU WISH TO LOSE WEIGHT . . .

DO MORE OF THIS	DO LESS OF THIS
Learn to notice and name your inner critic.	Treat whatever your inner critic says as the truth, for example: "Because of some defect, I can't lose weight."
Recognize that we all have a harsh inner critic, and all of us fail regularly at goals.	Believe that you alone are flawed and broken, for example: "I'm more flawed than others. I'm not as disciplined or as together as others. Others have got it easier than I have."
Acknowledge and make space for your inner critic. It's a natural part of you. You can't win a battle against it.	Fight your inner critic. Waste time trying to defeat it, for example: "I have to stop the criticism before I can start working toward my health goals."
Allow yourself to be motivated by an inner friend, that kind, accepting voice that gently encourages you.	Try to motivate yourself with a harsh critical voice. Be punishing rather than encouraging.

10.
SATISFYING YOUR TRUE HUNGER

We have declared peace on the battle with our bodies (Chapter 6). We have called a ceasefire in the war against our own emotions (Chapter 2). We have seen that although our mind can sometimes be an unreliable adviser and excessively critical (Chapter 4), we do not need to fight it. We can meet it on the battlefield with curiosity and kindness, and immediately the battle is over (Chapter 9). There is one final conflict that we must resolve and let go of—the battle between our competing desires.

Most of us experience desires that sometimes conflict. We want to give and care for others, but when we do this we sometimes forget to care for and comfort ourselves. We desire challenge but struggle to relax. We want to accomplish everything but seem to have too little energy and time. How do we handle these conflicts? Mostly we ignore them, or give up things that are important to us. However, there is one miracle drug that can seem to satisfy a good many of our desires, quickly and easily. That drug is called "food." It is one of the most powerful chemicals on earth. It can instantly give us comfort, stimulation, pleasure, a burst of energy, and relief from stress.

However, as you have figured out by now, there is a major downside to using food to get so many needs met. Non-hungry eating and neglecting self-care can take us away from our health goals, as in the figure on the next page.

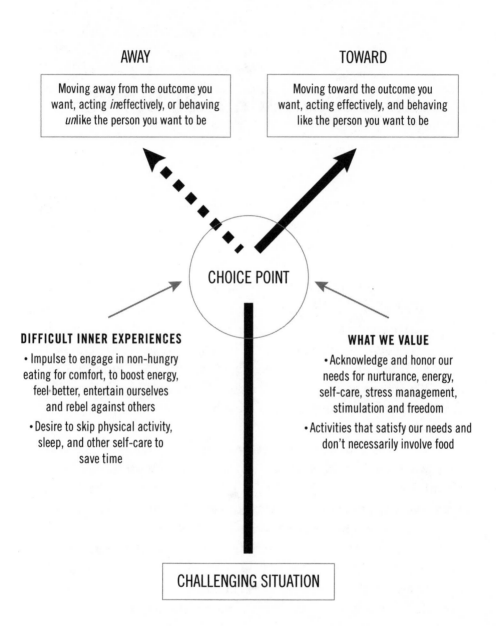

FIGURE 19: Does non-hungry eating give us what we truly value?

Non-hungry eating can easily lead us to gain weight, and make it harder to satisfy our other needs, as when lack of exercise and poor diet results in low energy and stress. We find ourselves in a strange conflict indeed: our own desire to get our needs met seems to be in conflict with our health needs. The key to ending this conflict is to first identify our non-hungry eating patterns and then to find new routines that allow us to get our needs met without overeating. Let's start by identifying the cues and rewards for our non-hungry eating. The quiz below will help you do just that.

ONE-MINUTE QUIZ: **WHAT DO YOU HUNGER FOR?**

Take this quiz to see how often you engage in non-hungry eating and what circumstances lead you to it.

CUE	DESIRED REWARD	EATING ROUTINE	HOW OFTEN DO YOU ENGAGE IN THIS EATING ROUTINE?				
			NEVER	RARELY	SOMETIMES	OFTEN	ALWAYS
Feeling lonely, insecure, or sad	Nurture	Eating comfort foods	0	1	2	3	4
Tiredness	Energy boost	Eating high-energy snacks or meals	0	1	2	3	4
Boredom	Stimulation	Eating as something fun to do	0	1	2	3	4
Feeling stressed	Stress relief	Eating fatty or sugary foods	0	1	2	3	4
Feeling time pressure	Saving time	Eating fast food or eating very quickly	0	1	2	3	4
Feeling pressured to eat the "right things" or look a certain way	Rebellion	Eating "disapproved of" foods to assert your independence	0	1	2	3	4
Procrastination	Distraction	Eating in order to avoid doing something	0	1	2	3	4
Feeling wronged and unable to obtain justice	Anger reduction	Eating to manage anger and/or frustration	0	1	2	3	4

If you tended to answer 2 or greater on the items (i.e., you scored between 16 and 32), then you often eat for reasons that have nothing to do with hunger. Look now at your favorite eating routine(s). What did you rate the highest?

Diet should never be denial

It is hard to live life denying ourselves what we want. That is true for diet too. When you've tried to lose weight in the past, how often have you been told what *not* to do. For example: "Don't eat too many carbohydrates/sweets/empty calories/fat?" There's nothing technically wrong with any of this advice, but it's not terribly inspiring, is it? Nobody wants their life to be about *not* doing things. No one says on their deathbed, "I wish I'd eaten less cheese."

Read Becky's story below and see if it rings any bells for you.

Becky's story: a not-quite-satisfying life

Becky lives a pretty normal life and tries to do the best she can, every day, for the people around her. With two children, a job and all the usual demands, Becky's life doesn't seem all that different from anyone else's, which is why Becky wonders about her weight, and why so many women seem to be thinner and fitter than her. *How do they do it?* she wonders. *Where do they find the time?*

Like most mothers, Becky begins her days early to stay on top of things. Not that she likes the early starts. She's exhausted all the time and curses the alarm every morning. But Becky is used to feeling tired, so she just tells herself to "suck it up and push on." By the time she's hung out two loads of washing, emptied the dishwasher, made the children's lunches and ironed her work clothes, everyone's awake and the morning chaos begins. Becky finally gets out the door and starts driving to work. Then she suddenly feels tired and realizes she hasn't eaten breakfast again. She gets something at the fast-food drive-through.

Throughout the day, Becky's energy goes up and down like a wave. She snacks to pick herself up before she has a proper meal. Then it's 5 p.m. and time to pick the kids up from school and manage the tennis lessons, swimming lessons and homework, cheer up her husband who's had a bad day at work, cook dinner, make sure the kids have their baths, and then get everyone off to bed.

Finally, at the end of the day, she finds peace and quiet. This is the moment she craves all day: everyone asleep and happy. This is her time now. She finally has some time and space to herself. She begins her nightly ritual by dimming the lights, turning on the TV and going to the fridge to find something she can enjoy "in peace and quiet."

Becky knows she *should* go to bed (because she always feels so tired) but this is *her* time, and there's no way she's giving that up for sleep. She settles in with her cheese and crackers, glass of wine and favorite show. Somewhere in the back of her mind, Becky thinks she should be eating celery or carrot sticks if she's still hungry, and certainly not eating a block of cheese, but this is her precious hour. Why should she give up enjoying the only moment she has to herself all day? "I'll start my diet and exercise tomorrow," she says to herself. But next morning, it all starts again.

Discovering new routines that satisfy your needs

We are faced with a dilemma. Because food temporarily satisfies many needs, cutting back on eating can lead us to feel unsatisfied in the short term. But if we are to lose weight, we need to reduce our psychological or non-hungry eating. The bind is clear: eating is our psychological support, yet to lose weight we need to take that support away. So what do we do?

The answer is to acknowledge our needs and honor them in a way that doesn't rely on food. And the very first step is to identify what our needs are. Once we know this, we can set about developing new routines that satisfy them. It all comes back to the habit loop. We've changed our cues, now we need to change our routines. We need to find a way to reduce psychological eating while still having our psychological needs met.

Figure 20 below illustrates a situation where the cue and the reward stay the same but the routine changes.

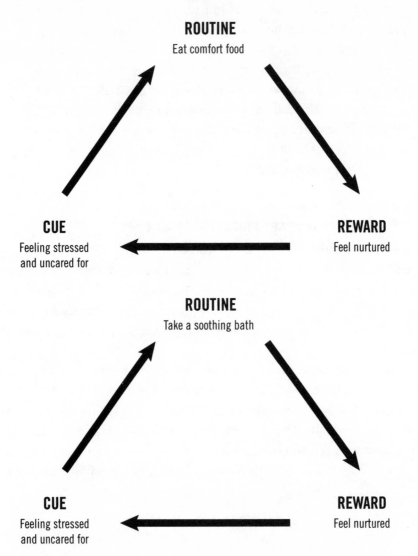

FIGURE 20: Altering the non-hungry eating routine in the habit loop

Nurturing yourself

We turn to food when we feel lonely, rejected, misunderstood or unacknowledged. We each have a different kind of comfort food. Here's how American author Ernest Hemingway described his comfort food in *A Moveable Feast*: "As I ate the oysters with their strong taste of the sea and their faint metallic taste that the cold white wine washed away, leaving only the sea taste and the succulent texture, and as I drank their cold liquid from each shell and washed it down with the crisp taste of wine, I lost the empty feeling and began to be happy and to make plans."

Sometimes we seek comfort in healthy foods, like chicken soup. Other times we seek comfort in chocolate, cookies, hamburgers and fries, pizza, fried eggs and cheese. Sometimes we eat all of these in the same day. Comfort foods are not inherently problematic. They only become a problem if and when eating them directly conflicts with our health goals. In this situation, we face a choice. Do we comfort ourselves with food or do we seek comfort elsewhere?

What else could we do to find comfort in our everyday life? There are many possibilities. We most often satisfy our need for nurture through connecting with other people. But if the people around us don't provide the nurture we need, it might be necessary for us to change our life in deeper ways. Chapter 2 helped you explore this, but if you feel the need, you can always re-read it and re-examine your core values. For now, let's spend time recognizing that there are ways to comfort and take care of ourselves that don't involve overeating. The possibilities are endless. Think about the last time you truly cared for yourself, by slowing down and asking yourself what you really needed in your life in that moment? Do you crave time to just "be," where you can slow down and just experience life as it is in each moment? What form of self-nurturance does this "being" time take for you? Would it be to take a mindful walk, where you were open to all the sensory experiences of sight, smell, sound, the ground under your feet, the trees, and birds in flight. Or could it be nurturing yourself by connecting with nature through gardening—feeling the earth between your fingers, smelling the flowers, watering the soil? If nature isn't your preferred form of self-nurturance, could you try something else, such as writing your thoughts and feelings in a beautiful journal, treating yourself to a coffee in a favorite coffee shop or buying a magazine you love but don't normally buy? And of course, even if you choose to forgo all those alternatives and instead choose to nurture yourself with a food treat, you can find a way to eat less of it and enjoy it more, using the mindfulness skills you learned in Chapter 7. Below are some examples of nurturing activities.

NURTURING ACTIVITIES THAT DON'T INVOLVE OVEREATING

- Turn off all electronic devices, unplug the phone
- Take a mindful walk with no destination in mind
- Take a hot bath
- Play something fun
- Do a hobby that is only for you
- Dance
- Keep a journal
- Light a fragrant candle
- Sit in the backyard and do nothing
- Have a mindful cup of tea
- Schedule time in your calendar for nurturing yourself
- Create something
- Exercise
- Reconnect with nature
- Stretch
- Meditate
- Sing
- Eat a small amount of a treat (buy the good stuff!)
- Find excuses to celebrate
- Get a massage
- Decorate
- Buy fresh flowers
- Get enough sleep
- Make a list of nurturing things to do, and schedule time to do them
- Watch a movie
- Join a book club
- Take a fun class
- Buy your favorite magazine
- Catch up with a friend
- Go fishing
- Lie on the grass and watch some clouds
- Go for a pedicure or manicure
- Play your favorite sport
- Play with a pet

Basically, it comes down to choice. We need to choose whether we want to engage in the same old eating routines or try something new. There's no right or wrong answer here.

SLEEP, ENERGY AND FOOD

Russ's energy boost

I spend a lot of time flying around Australia running workshops based on our ACT approach to weight loss. At the end of a full day of training, I'm exhausted. For many years, I'd go straight to my hotel room, flop on the bed and have a long nap. More often than not, though, I'd find that this nap, rather than making me feel refreshed, made me feel groggy and sluggish. So I started experimenting with an alternative approach. Even though I wanted to go to bed for a nap, I'd instead do some exercise: a brisk walk, a gym session or a swim in the pool. I found, to my surprise, that I actually felt more refreshed and energized by exercising than sleeping, and that I'd sleep much better that night.

If you eat when you're tired, you're not alone. Tiredness is one of the major reasons people give for eating too much food and the resultant weight gain. Sleeplessness seems to be the modern epidemic. Before World War I, adults slept an average of 8.7 hours a night. In 2008, adults were sleeping an average of only 6.7 hours a night. Indeed, sleep deprivation may be one of the biggest contributing factors to the obesity epidemic. One of the most important things you can do for yourself, therefore, is prioritize sleep. It's not something that's optional or can be cut. Your weight, and your very health, depend on it.

Even if you develop a foundation of good sleep, you may still at times eat high-calorie food to boost energy. If so, you might consider alternative energy-boosting routines. You might try drinking some tea, or getting up and moving around a bit. When you're tired, you might consider closing your eyes for a few minutes and taking a catnap. Or you might substitute fruit, yogurt, or soup for a high-calorie treat.

You may be surprised at what energizes you. Often, a bit of exercise or stretching or fresh air can do wonders. Smokers often go outside for a five-minute smoke break when they're tired. Non-smokers can learn something from this: the next time you're feeling tired, step outside for a five-minute walk or stretching session.

The take-home message of our author Russ's story above is that doing what comes naturally when you're tired is often self-defeating in the long term. Try doing something different, even if it seems counterintuitive.

More broadly, you might consider eating a diet that allows you to sustain your energy throughout the day. Perhaps the simplest way to do this is to lower the glycemic index (GI) of your foods, as described in Chapter 5. High-GI foods such as sweets, white rice, sweetened cereals and white bread give you a big hit of energy then leave you feeling depleted. That's when you're vulnerable to eating an unhealthy snack to boost your energy. Eat low-GI, slow-release food and you'll be better able to resist temptation.

Making time for you

Let's relate this advice to Becky's story from earlier in this chapter. We can see that Becky falls into these traps of eating for *energy* and to *self-nurture*. So how can she change these habits to support her weight-loss goals? The obvious problem is that she's not prioritizing her own needs, at any level, during her day. We all fall into this trap. Our author Ann, for example, says that this has happened to her. Read her story coming up and see how you relate to it.

There are many ways you can find time for yourself in your day. Sometimes that may mean using your assertiveness skills to draw up new boundaries and rules in your home. For example, you might set aside a certain time each day that is just for you and what you want to do. Or, at work, you could draw some new boundaries by requesting a regular, uninterrupted lunch break every day, or even negotiate to start work an hour earlier or later each day. Once you've found "your time," you need to commit to keeping this a *health non-negotiable* and weave your duties and life around it. Just with all health behaviors you choose to commit to, placing health first and duties second feels like an impossible task at the beginning, but it can be done. It just comes down to creating new habits. And once new health habits are formed, weight loss is not far away.

Ann's "me" time

I felt like I couldn't possibly find any time in the day to devote to myself, when the needs of my family and work were so great. I developed the habit of placing everyone else's needs before my own, only to realize I'd run out of time by the end of the day to give anything back to myself. It was starting to make me feel quite resentful and agitated, which then began to have a negative influence on my relationships with my husband and kids. Initially, I tried to fix things by sacrificing essentials, like sleep, to give myself time and space. I also started giving myself small but regular chocolate treats after dinner each night to help me tolerate the post-dinner clean-up. These habits became my daily reward. And my weight started to rise.

So what did I do to change these habits? I started by prioritizing my health needs, then fitting the rest of my life and duties around these. First, I targeted my sleep. Clearly I was tired and needed more hours of sleep than I was getting. So I developed a principle never to go to bed any later than 9:30 p.m. every night. This is one of my health non-negotiables. Initially it felt like I was missing out on me time at night, but when I stayed committed, I realized my increased sleep had a ripple effect on the rest of my life. It led to massive improvements in my mood and agitation levels, and I found that it eventually led to *more* time out for myself, not less.

Once I began prioritizing my sleep, my next health non-negotiable was making time during the day that was mine and mine alone. I realized that unless I did this, I would continue to want to reward myself with food or deprive myself of sleep. So, I decided to allocate one hour a day to myself. You're probably thinking there's no way you would be able to fit an extra hour in for yourself during your day. That's what I thought, too, but believe me when I say it's possible. It's all about the skill of placing your health priorities *first* then working your other duties around them. I found it incredibly hard to start giving myself an hour a day, but it was necessary for my health, wellbeing and relationships. I also knew that, ultimately, it would help my weight loss too.

So I began to take time out in the morning, before the day began. This change also required me to negotiate and assert myself with my husband so he could support me taking this time. It meant he had to step up and prepare the children's breakfast and so on while I had "my time." He was willing to support my new habit. So, with my precious hour every day, I actually chose to take a slow, mindful walk. Although I could have done many different things with my time, this regular walk was the time for me to nurture and give back to myself.

I haven't looked back. My health non-negotiables are a part of my life. And surprisingly, I now have no urgency to stay up late for "my time," because I get it in the morning. And, the nice thing is, because I'm going to bed earlier, I don't mind getting up earlier. The other bonus is that I don't feel as compelled to reward myself with treats after dinner because I already feel I've had my reward with my morning time. And my weight *has* gone down.

Managing stress

Our bodies are exquisitely designed to manage physical stress. Imagine a large dog approaches you, snarling and showing its teeth. You realize it's about to attack, and that's when your brain triggers the release of hormones and other chemicals into the bloodstream that ready you either to run away or to fight it off: the famous fight-or-flight response we discussed in Chapter 7. Your large muscles tense ready for action, your reflexes speed up and you become hyper-alert. Your heart rate and blood pressure increase, and the body systems not needed to deal with the immediate threat, such as your digestive, immune and reproductive systems, shut down. In other words, every part of you prepares for immediate action.

Action is needed in harsh, life-threatening environments, to find shelter from a storm, run from a wolf, scavenge for water, hunt a buffalo, fight off your enemy, and so on. But most of us don't live in those sorts of environments any more. We live in relative safety and comfort, in houses that protect us from the elements, far away from dangerous animals. Why, then, do we get so stressed out? It's because we face so many psychological threats that can't be solved by physical action. For example, if we learn that someone is talking negatively about us at work, we know it's not a good idea to physically attack that person. Nor is it easy to flee the person if we need to keep our job. So we react to that person the same way we would to a snarling animal: our body goes into fight-or-flight mode. We're hotwired for immediate physical action, yet we can't physically act. This physical state of racing heart, tense muscles, agitation, speediness and restlessness is what we usually refer to when we talk about feeling stressed.

We experience hundreds of psychological stresses every day—worries, insecurities, regrets, frustrations, disappointments and irritations—and we can't simply attack them or run away. No wonder most of us experience chronic stress.

And as it happens, chronic stress has a lot to do with weight control. If the energy mobilized by the fight-or-flight response is not used, it gets stored as fat around the belly. Furthermore, when we're feeling stressed, we prefer food that's high in sugar and/or fat. This goes for the authors of this book, too: Joseph finds nothing more soothing after a stressful day than a greasy hamburger while Russ prefers chocolate and Ann cheese. Others may prefer doughnuts, toast and butter, or potato chips. We each have our stress-reduction foods of choice.

Our challenge, then, is to find ways to manage our stress with routines that don't involve eating high-calorie foods. The good news is, there are scientifically supported methods to manage stress. Probably the single best method is exercise. If stress causes our body to prepare for physical action, the natural way to react to that stress is to engage in physical action. Exercise is a way of giving our stressed body exactly what it needs.

Many people groan when we mention exercise: they immediately think of it as tedious, boring, painful or too hard. But exercise doesn't have to be long, or involve going to the gym. It could be something as simple as taking a 10-minute walk, which research shows is enough to reduce tension. It's worth thinking about creative ways to bring exercise into your life and use it as a substitute for stress-driven eating. The great thing about exercise is, not only does it help us with weight loss, it protects us from cancer, depression and heart disease. How's that for value?

PRACTICING MINDFULNESS TO REDUCE STRESS

Another scientifically supported way to reduce stress is through mindfulness practice (see Chapter 7) or meditation. Again, we don't have to meditate every day to reap the benefits, nor do we need to meditate for long periods of time. If you're feeling stressed, and know you're about to eat something unhealthy, you can try simply meditating on your breathing for five minutes and see if that helps (see Chapter 7). Indeed, even doing this for just one minute can make a big difference. Chapter 7 also offers concrete ways to weave mindfulness into your everyday life.

THE TRUE GOAL OF STRESS REDUCTION

Whatever stress-reducing habit you choose, it's important to remember that our ultimate goal is not stress reduction but to make our life rich, full and meaningful. And as we discussed in Chapter 1, acting on our values to make our life richer and fuller can generate stress. If we wish to build loving relationships, for example, we open ourselves to the stress associated with rejection, loss, frustration, disappointment and the inevitable conflicts that occur in even the best of relationships. Similarly, if we choose to pursue meaningful life goals, we encounter the stress of failure. And if we wish to exercise, we will inevitably stress our bodies (but, of course, this is healthy stress).

The point is, stress—and the uncomfortable thoughts and feelings that go with it—is an important part of life. So whatever stress-reduction routine you decide on, make sure it's making your life better, not worse. For example, drinking three bottles of wine a night might be an effective means of temporarily reducing stress, but it won't be good for your health or relationships.

Combating boredom

We often want to take a break from work or a tedious activity or simply to procrastinate. It's natural to make these breaks about eating. It's the kind of break we can justify: we have to eat, don't we? There's an easy way to find out if you're using food as a distraction: substitute some enjoyable or interesting routine for the food break and see if that satisfies you. This might be taking a walk, playing a video game, reading a magazine, checking emails, drinking tea, or doing some activity you love.

What happens when you do this new activity instead of eating? Does the urge to eat pass, or do you feel genuinely hungry? If the former, you can substitute the new routine for your procrastination eating. If, however, you still genuinely feel hungry, maybe it really is time to eat.

But again, take a moment to check in with your body. What do you notice in your mouth? And what do you notice in your stomach? Ask yourself, "Is my stomach genuinely wanting food or is it just that my mouth wants flavor, texture, something to do?" If the latter, maybe the best option is to drink an herbal tea, chew some sugar-free gum or suck on a sugar-free mint.

Joseph's angry eating

When I lost 20 pounds, everybody suddenly started offering me their opinions about my body: "Oh, you were a little pudgy before" or "You look different in your jeans" or "You've lost weight but you still have love handles." I was upset. When did my body become open to public discussion? And if people judged me as too fat before I lost the weight, what would happen if I put the weight back on? They'd judge me again. My first reaction to these comments about my body was to rebel by eating whatever high-calorie food I wanted to eat.

Dealing with anger

Now we come to one of the deepest psychological triggers to eat: anger. Sometimes we eat to give people the middle finger and let them know they don't control our body. As Joseph's story above shows, anger can be like eating rat poison and hoping the rat will die.

A second kind of angry eating occurs when we're being treated unfairly and we can't seem to assert our rights. We feel powerless. Eating is one form of assertion. Eating says, "I deserve consideration. I have rights."

We do have rights. We have the right not to be judged. We have the right to be treated fairly. And, of course, we have the right to eat whatever we want and be as large as we wish to be. But we need to ask ourselves whether this angry eating helps us assert those rights or just gets us further entangled in anger and self-defeating patterns of behavior.

When anger with someone triggers our eating, we become more involved with that person. In other words, we give them more power and influence over us, not less. When we face pressure from people, or society in general, we have three possible responses:

1. CONFORM TO WHAT OTHERS WANT FOR US

This could involve trying to look like an anorexic fashion model or a buffed-up bodybuilder.

2. REBEL AGAINST WHAT PEOPLE WANT AND DO THE OPPOSITE

If, for example, our mom suggests we shouldn't eat so much, we could promptly double our serving size, to show her who's in control. Of course, sometimes these acts of rebellion work against us; we're fighting back against that inner dictator (see Chapter 4) who's always telling us what we should, shouldn't, can or can't eat.

3. FIND THE MIDDLE WAY

We need to choose the path that takes us in a direction we wish to go, but is neither conformity nor rebellion. Rather it's conscious living, based on our core values.

At times that middle path may mean losing some weight because it's personally important to us, or because it gives us energy and vitality to invest in other meaningful areas of our life, or because we care about our health and wellbeing—rather than losing weight because other people want us to or think we should. At other times, that middle path involves choosing not to lose weight because we're at peace with our current size and shape. Choosing not to diet at these times isn't an act of rebellion or righteous indignation or showing them who's boss. It's simply an affirmation of our values.

The key is to be guided by your own inner values rather than conformity to society's expectations or angry rebellion against those expectations.

SUMMARY: IF YOU WISH TO LOSE WEIGHT . . .

DO MORE OF THIS	DO LESS OF THIS
Learn to recognize your non-hungry eating routines.	Assume you eat only when you're hungry.
Find new ways, other than non-hungry eating, to satisfy your needs.	Deny your needs and deprive yourself.

11.
ENHANCE YOUR LIFE

The previous chapter showed you that there are many activities, other than eating, that help you meet your needs. This chapter will help you to identify the activities that are most likely to bring you lasting fulfillment. There's a wealth of good scientific research that addresses this topic, and it basically tells us fulfillment in life arises from activities that satisfy our basic needs. These include activities that provide us with:

1. safety, security and sustenance
2. positive relationships
3. challenge
4. enjoyment.

So let's now examine our own lives with this research in mind. Here are four questions you can ask of any activity you engage in:

1. Does this activity provide safety, security or sustenance?
2. Does this activity help me develop positive relationships with others?
3. Does this activity challenge me?
4. Is this activity enjoyable?

If you can answer yes to at least one of these questions, the activity will be life-enhancing (so long as you do it in a flexible way, not with a fused, rigid mindset). However, it's unlikely that any one activity you choose will allow you to say yes to all four questions.

Let's now look a bit closer at each of these needs: why they are so important to your life. Later, we will ask you to consider how your health and other life goals satisfy the needs.

1. Does this activity provide safety, security or sustenance?

Food, water and shelter are our most basic needs. If we don't have enough to eat or drink, or we're not safe from threats, then we won't be able to do much else effectively. On top of that, we need enough money to live. We need to surround ourselves with people who help us and care about us, and don't neglect or mistreat us. And we need to eat healthily and exercise regularly to sustain our body and prevent disease.

So if our current activity involves buying things or eating things that we don't really need, our answer to the question above—*Does this activity provide safety, security or sustenance?*—will typically be "no." We might call these activities *empty strivings*. They fill up our time but provide us with no vital sustenance, and no meaningful safety or security. The more we let go of empty strivings, the more time we have for genuinely life-enhancing pursuits. In the realm of health, perhaps some of your health goals do not sustain you, such as when you go on a starvation diet, or some fad diet that requires you to eat strange food combinations or eliminate entire food groups. Fulfilling health goals are the ones that help us to sustain our energy and vitality during the day.

2. Does this activity help me develop positive relationships with others?

Humans need each other. If you doubt this, take a look around you at all the wondrous things you use but probably didn't make: the furniture, the windows, the art on the wall, the computer, the TV. Think of the electricity running through your house, supplied by a group of people you've probably never met. Think of your meal tonight and how you didn't have to hunt for it, and the fuel in your car and how you didn't have to dig it up from the earth and process it. Our interdependence is so complete we don't even notice it.

We need each other. When we're cut off from other people, we become depressed and sick. Indeed, one of the worst tortures ever devised is solitary confinement. Research suggests that our happiness level fluctuates a great deal throughout the day. And when are we typically most unhappy? When we're alone! And when are we typically most contented? When we're with genuine friends. Ask anybody, "Deep down inside, what's most important in your life?" and they'll almost always answer something like "my friends" or "my children" or "my family."

Given relationships are so important, it's strange that we spend so little time actively and consciously developing them. We often spend much more time shopping, developing our career, working and doing other tasks. The one sure way to improve our wellbeing is to spend more time improving our relationships. So how can your health-related goals help with this? Can you make healthy eating a regular part of socializing? Can you find ways to make exercising something you share with your friends and loved ones? For example, when Russ goes out to dinner with friends, he often asks if they'd like to go for a half-hour walk before or afterwards. Joseph has played tennis with his friends every Thursday for the last 12 years. Ann meets one of her closest friends once a week to share a training session and catch-up afterwards.

3. Does this activity challenge me?

When life seems overly busy and stressful, most of us tend to wonder if we'd be happier winning the lottery and spending the rest of our days in retirement, perhaps relaxing on the beach. Does that sound appealing to you? While there's definitely a place for relaxation in our lives, research suggests that we'd actually be pretty miserable if all we did was lie around.

The most fulfilled people are those who regularly challenge themselves and get actively involved in meaningful activities. These people don't necessarily engage in huge challenges like jumping out of a plane, but they do engage in everyday challenges such as gardening, reading books, bowling, teaching, cooking a good meal, playing games, exercising and working.

Of course, not all challenge is good. If something is too challenging, we may feel stressed, frustrated or anxious, and therefore not enjoy it. And if it's not challenging enough, we'll experience boredom or apathy.

The key is to find the right balance between challenge and our ability to handle the challenge: we want to stretch ourselves, but not so far that we feel we can't cope. When the challenge is equal to our resources, we often experience a state called *flow*, which involves effortless concentration, absorption and enjoyment. In this state, we lose track of time, and nothing else seems to matter other than the activity itself.

The flow experience is likely to occur when we're engaged in hobbies, sports and games, or meaningful social interactions. However, it's unlikely to occur when we're engaged in passive activities, such as watching boring TV shows. Nevertheless, the average person spends about four times as much free time watching TV than engaging in hobbies and sports. Why do we engage in so many passive activities if they don't bring us joy? The problem is one of inertia.

Doing something challenging takes initial effort before it becomes enjoyable. Exercise reduces stress and promotes wellbeing, but we don't achieve those benefits until *after* we exercise. *Before* we exercise, we often have to do a number of things that aren't intrinsically rewarding, such as get out of bed early, drive to the gym and take time away from other things. Before exercising, it seems like too much effort and we want to take the easy, passive option. Maybe we'll watch the morning news or just stay in bed and sleep a bit longer. Unfortunately, the more we choose the easy option, the more unfulfilled we tend to become. This bears repeating: fulfilled people tend to take the active option, whether that be exercising, pursuing a hobby or working on a project that is personally meaningful.

In this book you've learned three techniques that are useful for overcoming inertia. First, we can turn our activity into a habit, so that we do it automatically (see Chapter 8). Second, if we feel like we don't want to do something because we are "too tired," "too stressed" or it's "too boring" or "too hard," we can use the approach described in Chapters 2 and 3: make room for those thoughts and feelings and do the activity anyway, even though we don't feel like it in that moment. Essentially, we embrace this "golden rule":

**The actions of wellbeing come first;
the feelings of wellbeing come later.**

In the realm of exercise, willingness often involves feeling tired or unmotivated, and even so, persisting with our exercise routine.

The third technique for overcoming inertia is to use the defusion and self-compassion skills described in Chapters 4 and 9. Remember, the reasons our minds give us to avoid exercise or eat unwisely are not physical barriers that stop us (see Chapter 5). They're neither more nor less than words inside our heads that continually come and go. If we notice them mindfully, using the techniques covered in Chapter 5, they can't push us around and dictate what we do.

4. Is this activity enjoyable and/or personally important to me or am I just doing it for other people?

We like to be the authors of our lives, and most of us hate feeling controlled by others. For example, imagine you love playing games; you do it all the time without anybody asking or telling you to. Now imagine someone offers to pay you real money to keep on playing those very same games. In this scenario, do you think you'd spend more time or less time playing? Most people imagine they'd play more: *"You're paying me to do something I'd happily do for nothing? Of course I'd do more of it!"* But research actually reveals the opposite is true. If you get paid to play, you're likely to play *less*. That's right. Once money is involved, playing the game is your job. In other words, you feel like you're being forced to play. It doesn't feel so much fun any more. There's a sense of *obligation* about it; you're doing it to please others (the folks who are paying your wages). You've lost your sense of control.

In general, more fulfilled people have a strong sense of control in their life. So the more we do things because of pressure from others, or fear of their disapproval, or worries about what they might think of us, the less our sense of control in life. And in the realm of dieting and exercise, it's all too easy for this to happen; we need to be on the lookout for it. Our sense of control increases when we find our own internal reasons for committing to healthy action; not when we try to please others or avoid their disapproval.

EXERCISE: **ARE MY GOALS LIFE-ENHANCING?**

Write down your key life goals on the left. Make sure you list some goals related to health and goals not directly related to health. Rate from 0 (does not satisfy this need) to 10 (strongly satisfies this need).

NEEDS

LIFE GOALS OR ACTIVITIES	BRINGS SAFETY, SECURITY OR SUSTENANCE	DEVELOPS POSITIVE RELATIONSHIPS	CHALLENGES ME	GIVES ME ENJOYMENT

I do these activities now:

I would like to start doing these activities:

Take a look at what you wrote above and consider some of these questions. Are you getting all your needs met from your activities? Do all your activities tend to be for one thing (e.g., safety or challenge)? Do you spend way too much time on one activity, and not enough on other activities? What health-related activities might you do more of, in order to get your needs met?

SUMMARY: IF YOU WISH TO LOSE WEIGHT . . .

DO MORE OF THIS	DO LESS OF THIS
Pursue health goals because you enjoy them, or because they are personally meaningful to you.	Pursue goals because that is what you feel you "should" or "must" do.
Find ways to challenge yourself. Compete against others, or against your own best scores and times.	Avoid challenge as "too stressful."
Eat food that gives you sustained energy and health.	Sacrifice your diet for weight loss, eat food that has few nutrients, or starve yourself in order to lose weight.
If socializing is important to you, find ways to spend time with others and pursue your health goals, make health a social activity.	Don't socialize until you have lost weight, wait until your weight is at the "right" level to start living.

12.
FINDING YOUR FAITH AND COURAGE

This chapter brings our journey to a close, and starts us on a new journey into our unknown future. We have explored how we can live mindfully in the moment and make values-based choices. No matter how tough our life has been, no matter how many times we have failed at our goals, we have a chance at redemption in each new moment. Every second gives us the opportunity to fully engage with and appreciate the things we care about. The key is to show up to life with faith in ourselves and the courage to commit.

FAITH VERSUS REASON

What is the difference between faith and reason? Well, think about something you did that was hard, and you weren't sure you could do it, but you went ahead and had a go at doing it anyway. That is what we call an "act of faith," or a "faith move." You didn't know you would succeed—but you "had faith in yourself"; you relied on yourself to do what needed doing. Note we're not talking about "faith" in any religious sense. The word "faith" comes from the Latin "fides," which also means "trust," "fidelity," "reliability" and "truth." So an act of faith in yourself means trusting yourself, being true to yourself; this is what we mean by a "faith move."

Now think about a time when you motivated yourself to do something by thinking it through carefully and coming up with reasons for why you could plausibly succeed at it. That is a "reason move"; you reasoned yourself into it.

Our reasoning mind has its limitations, as we discussed in Chapters 4 and 5. It tends to be excessively negative (to help us survive) and it tends to be extremely convincing. While it can be successful at motivating us, by giving us lots of "good reasons" to do something important, far more often it *demotivates* us by coming up with all the reasons *not* to do something important. Just about every time we try to do something hard or important, our mind generates doubts: it comes up with all sorts of reasons why we can't do it, shouldn't do it, or shouldn't even have to do it. If we always allowed these doubts to dominate our actions, we would probably be unable to do anything remotely challenging in life.

The reasoning mind is often most unhelpful when we are trying to motivate ourselves to do something new: stepping out of our comfort zone into a challenging situation with an uncertain outcome. For example, suppose you are trying to lose weight, or keep it off, but you have never successfully done this before—at least, not for long. Your mind is likely to reason along these lines: "Because I've always failed at this in the past, I'm naturally going to fail again now; so there's no point even trying to lose weight or keep it off; I'm doomed to failure." And, if you buy into that reasoning, what are the odds that you will lose weight? We would guess zero!

There are many areas in life where we just don't have good solid evidence that we can succeed at something. For example, if you have had a string of bad relationships, your reasoning mind might plausibly conclude that you are "always unlucky in love—so there's no point in trying any more." Should you let this type of reasoning control your actions; give up just because your mind likes to speak to you this way? Or would it be more life-enhancing to make the "faith move"—to assume that if you persist long enough and hard enough and vary your strategies enough, then finding a loving partner is possible?

There are times when we have to sidestep our reasoning minds and have faith in our ability to change and grow. We need to assume something is possible even though we don't know that it is for certain. This faith move is extremely difficult. It often means doing something when your mind is screaming at you, "Give up. It's useless. You'll fail. You're wasting your time!" The faith move is an act of great courage, as we will discuss below. It is a choice you can make no matter what your mind is telling you. Thus, to some extent, it liberates you from your mind and increases your freedom to pursue the things you care about.

Now, we consider two questions of faith we need to ask ourselves (again and again).

1. CAN YOU ACCEPT YOURSELF ON FAITH?

Can you start the rest of your life with the assumption that you are already whole, complete and good enough? If you do make this faith move, you'll notice your reasoning mind will try to convince you to give it up. That's okay. This is a faith move, which means you can make it no matter what your mind tells you.

Let's look at the pragmatics of accepting yourself on faith. If you assumed that you are already whole, complete, and good enough, what might you start doing?

If, in contrast, you assume you are somehow broken and not good enough, how might you act? Which assumption/faith move is better for your life?

2. CAN YOU ACCEPT ON FAITH THAT YOU CAN IMPROVE YOUR LIFE?

Again this leads to a practical question. If you assume improvement is possible, what might you do? If you assume it is not possible, what might you do instead?

A NEW FORM OF SUCCESS

If we accept on faith that success is possible, we must now answer the question: what is success? Society has a clear answer. Success means achieving our goals. Society considers us successful if we lose a certain amount of weight, get a promotion, earn lots of money, marry someone wonderful, buy a lovely house, or win a contest. We can check those goals off the list: done! And of course, from this perspective on success, if we don't achieve the goal we've failed.

From the youngest age, we're taught to perform well in exams and achieve good marks. People who win at sports get all the awards, while the person who finishes in fourth place goes unrecognized. At work we're encouraged to achieve key performance indicators, such as selling a certain number of products. We're so obsessed with achieving outcomes we fail to notice that there's another way to define success.

Values-based success is not defined by achieving our goals. Values-based success is defined purely and simply by how well we are living in accordance with our values. We are successful whenever we act consistently with our own values, no matter how small that action may be, no matter if it's invisible or uninteresting or even disapproved of by others. Say, for example, your goal is to get someone at work to treat you well. You act respectfully and kindly toward this person, but despite your best efforts, they continue to treat you badly and stab you in the back. In terms of goal-based success, you've failed! You didn't achieve your goal: you didn't get this person to treat you well. However, in terms of values-based success, you've been highly successful: you acted consistently with your values of kindness and respect.

Thus, when seeking to improve your health, it's important to focus on values-based rather than goal-based success. This is because we actually don't have that much day-to-day control over things like our weight, blood pressure or immune function. The body is extremely complex and unpredictable. For example, have you ever had a week where you stuck perfectly to your diet, exercised a lot and then got on the scales only to discover you'd gained weight? How frustrating is that? Again, in terms of goal-based success, you've failed! But in terms of values-based success, did you fail? No way! You were highly successful, because you acted consistently with your value of self-care. If you keep acting consistently with your self-care values, eventually you will achieve more of the outcomes you want, such as improved health.

Another important feature of values-based success is that it occurs when we honor *all* our values, not just those related to weight loss. Indeed, research suggests that when we engage in values that aren't directly related to weight loss, we're actually most likely to experience weight loss. This is great news. It means we don't have to wait until the weight comes off to start connecting with people, having fun and influencing the world.

Our time is now.

QUIET COURAGE

The word "courage" comes from the Latin word "cor," which means "heart." So courage basically means doing what is in your heart. Most people think of courage in dramatic overtones, as when someone jumps from a bridge into freezing water to save a drowning child. But there's another, quieter form of courage, which is often invisible to other people. It's the courage to say yes to what we care about. And we need to exercise this type of courage almost every single day of our life.

Commitment to living by our values is an act of quiet courage. If we seek success, we risk failure. If we seek connection with others, we risk rejection and disappointment. If we love someone, we risk losing them. Even joyful moments have their sorrow, because we know that every joyful moment must pass.

There's no shelter from the natural pain of life. We've all sought shelter by hiding in our house and making no commitments. But that never works. It just makes us feel sadness and regret, because we know we've wasted our time.

We need quiet courage to live well in this world. We need to practice saying yes to risk in the service of the things we care most about. The courageous "yes" gets easier when we practice the skills outlined in this book. We can learn to defuse or step back from our mind when it is criticizing us and telling us we're going to fail, and giving us reasons to give up.

We can't turn our mind off or escape it—at least not for long. What we can do is learn to notice mindfully that thoughts come and go. We might notice our mind judging us as not good enough, for example, and then notice a leaf falling from a tree. We can see that both events are the same, both are passing, both will happen again. Self-judgments will happen, leaves will fall. But neither self-judgment nor falling leaves need stop us from living a rich and meaningful life.

SUMMARY: IF YOU WISH TO LOSE WEIGHT . . .

DO MORE OF THIS	DO LESS OF THIS
Have faith in your ability to change.	Think you are in any way incomplete or deficient.
Recognize the limitations of your reasoning mind.	Focus exclusively on weight loss—honoring other values will help you achieve your goals.
Act consistently with your own values.	Elevate goal-based success above value-based success.

THE SEVEN-WEEK WEIGHT ESCAPE BOOT CAMP

The seven-week boot camp gives you a chance to practice all of the skills taught in the book. We hope you find it useful.

WEEK 1: GETTING CLEAR ON YOUR VALUES

This exercise has two parts:

1. Explore and rate the principles that guide your life
2. Spot the values that underpin your actions

PART 1: EXPLORE AND RATE THE PRINCIPLES THAT GUIDE YOUR LIFE

This exercise will help you to take a detailed look at your guiding principles. Please take your time and rate each principle according to the following.

Importance: 0 = unimportant to me; 9 = extremely important to me.
(This is what you find important, not necessarily what others find important.)

Success: 0 = not at all successful; 9 = highly successful.
(This is how successful you feel you've been in living consistently by your principles.)

PRINCIPLE	IMPORTANCE	SUCCESS
1. Connecting with nature		
2. Gaining wisdom		
3. Creating beauty (in any domain, including arts, dancing, gardening)		
4. Promoting justice and caring for the weak		
5. Being loyal to friends, family, and/or my group		
6. Being honest		
7. Helping others		
8. Being sexually desirable		
9. Having genuine and close friends		
10. Having relationships involving love and affection		
11. Being ambitious and hard working		
12. Being competent and effective		
13. Having a sense of accomplishment and making a lasting contribution		
14. Having an exciting life		
15. Having a life filled with adventure		
16. Having a life filled with novelty and change		
17. Being physically fit		
18. Eating healthy foods		
19. Engaging in sporting activities		
20. Acting consistently with my religious faith and beliefs		
21. Being at one with God		
22. Showing respect for tradition		
23. Being spiritual		
24. Being self-disciplined and resisting temptation		
25. Meeting my obligations		
26. Maintaining the safety and security of my loved ones		
27. Making sure to repay favors and not be indebted to people		
28. Being safe from danger		

PRINCIPLE	IMPORTANCE	SUCCESS
29. Being wealthy		
30. Having authority, being in charge		
31. Having influence over people		
32. Having a leisurely life		
33. Enjoying food and drink		
34. Being sexually active		
35. Being creative		
36. Being self-sufficient		
37. Being curious, discovering new things		
38. Figuring out things, solving problems		
39. Striving to be a better person		
40. Enjoying music, art, and/or drama		
41. Designing things		
42. Teaching others		
43. Resolving disputes		
44. Building and repairing things		
45. Working with my hands		
46. Organizing things		
47. Engaging in clearly defined work		
48. Researching things		
49. Competing with others		
50. Being admired by many people		
51. Acting with courage		
52. Caring for others		
53. Accepting others as they are		
54. Working on practical tasks		
55. Seeking pleasure		
56. Being attractive		

PART 2: **SPOT THE VALUES THAT UNDERPIN YOUR ACTIONS**

Now we would like you to look at your responses from Part 1. We want you to identify principles you find important but do not feel that you have been successful at. We want you to particularly focus on things you want to improve on.

a) Write down five principles you find important and want to improve on

1. _____
2. _____
3. _____
4. _____
5. _____

b) Identify the underlying value to those principles

For each principle, ask yourself two questions:

1. What are some example actions you might engage in to put this principle into play?
2. Why are you doing those actions? Think of the sort of person *you* want to be.

Here is an example:

Principle: Accepting others as they are
Actions: Let my friend know it is okay to feel anxious; do not criticize for minor things.
Find the value. I want to be the sort of person who: is a loving, supportive friend.

Now write about your principles, and do your best to spot the value. Do not worry about doing this exercise exactly right. Your effort is the most important thing. This exercise will help you to identify the kind of person you want to be.

Principle 1: _____
Actions:

_____
_____

Find the value. I want to be the sort of person who:

_____
_____

Principle 2: _____
Actions:

_____
_____

Find the value. I want to be the sort of person who:

_____
_____

Principle 3: _____
Actions:

_____
_____

Find the value. I want to be the sort of person who:

_____
_____

Principle 4: _____
Actions:

_____
_____

Find the value. I want to be the sort of person who:

_____
_____

Principle 5: _____
Actions:

_____
_____

Find the value. I want to be the sort of person who:

_____
_____

Spotting the value is key to everything. It will help you to stay on course and committed even when you fail at your goals. For example, you might have the value "engaging in healthy behaviors." Sometimes you won't act consistently with this value (e.g., you might binge on choco- late). However, no matter how many times you leave your valued path, your value is still yours to claim. It is not cancelled out by failure. You can keep committing to it. Nobody can take it away from you.

WEEK 2: DEVELOPING YOUR O.W.L. SKILLS

Introducing the O.W.L.

Now we will introduce you to an acronym that combines the core skills we have been working on in this book: O.W.L., which stands for Ob- serving, Willingness and Living your values. This acronym will be help- ful when you are in situations where you need to take a mindful pause and make a choice associated with your health and weight-loss journey. Let's now take a closer look at the O.W.L. skills.

OBSERVING

Another word for observing is "mindfulness," which is the main word we've used throughout the book. This skill involves using breathing tech- niques to help us pay attention to something with curiosity. Observing helps you to respond effectively to your own feelings and thoughts. Self- doubt does not need to stop you from succeeding. Fear does not need to block you from finding friends or love. Observing lets you take a step back from your own difficult feelings and choose the most effective path. Observing also helps you to spot your strengths and use them to get more of what you want in life.

WILLINGNESS

Willingness is most similar to courage. It is about choosing to do some- thing that is important to you, even if it means some distress along the way. Are you willing to have self-doubt in order to give a speech? Are you willing to feel a little fear in order to attempt conversation? Can you have boredom "visit you" and still stay committed to exercising? Each time you answer yes to a question like this you are choosing to "be willing." You are willingly having difficult feelings in order to act effectively. It takes courage to risk fear, sadness, embarrassment, or anger. However, this does not mean you should always be willing. There are some things that just aren't important enough for you to be willing to do. We choose to be willing only for those things we deeply care about.

LIVING YOUR VALUES

Living your way means discovering what matters and living according to this. We call this living your values. When we talk about values, we mean what is most important to you, not what is important to other people. What do you want in life? How would you like to live? Values are your compass. Without them, you can wander aimlessly.

Using your O.W.L. skills to cope with tough situations

Below is a simple exercise that you can do in your day-to-day life. It can be especially useful when you are struggling to make a value-enhancing decision. We recommend you copy out this exercise and keep it in your wallet or purse as a reminder. We recommend you do it for the next week, perhaps first thing in the morning.

EXERCISE: **O.W.L.**

Observing: Focus on your breath, then observe inside (what am I feeling?). Expand the observing to the outside (what am I doing? what is around me?).

Willingness: Willingness means choosing to do something that is important to you, even if it means having some distress along the way. Are you willing to have the distress you observed in order to make a valued choice? If yes, allow the distress to just be. Notice it. Breathe in and around it. Make space.

Living your values: In this moment, I will _____ (think of the kind of quality you want to display in this moment; e.g., persist, be disciplined, be kind, build health, express friendship, love, have fun).

We begin O.W.L. by focusing on the breath. The breath brings us into the present moment, where we are able to make a choice—whether to move toward or away from what we care about. You can play around with the kind of breathing exercise you want to do (see Chapter 7). For example, here are three variations of observing your breath:

- Breathe slowly. Inhale for four seconds then pause. Exhale for four seconds and pause again.
- Just notice the breath. Every breath is just right.
- Count each outbreath until you get to 10 and then start at 1 again.

This stage can be as brief or as long as you want. It is the critical pause, where you will find your awareness and freedom. It can undermine the power of unhelpful thoughts and put you and your values in charge. Once you have finished observing the breath, you shift your attention to observing your inner experiences. This will create a wise space between you and your difficult feelings and thoughts, what we called "defusion" in Chapter 3. Then you expand your awareness to what you are doing.

WEEK 3: FREEING YOURSELF FROM PRESSURE

People close to us and society at large are often pressuring us to act a certain way, look a certain way and eat a certain way. It is difficult to hear our own voice in the midst of all this pressure and judgment from others. Sometimes we react badly to pressure, as when we deliberately rebel against it, even when such rebellion is against our best interests (e.g., eating too much just to defy our judgmental mom). Sometimes we conform to pressure but then we soon become demotivated and stop doing the things we care about. This week we will explore a way of getting free from pressure and basing our choices on our own values, not merely on rebellion or conformity. This week will also give you a chance to practice your O.W.L. skills so that you can learn how to respond to pressure effectively. More specifically we are going to invite you to:

OBSERVING

Notice the things you do that you feel pressured to do, and the thoughts, feelings and sensations that are linked to it.

WILLINGNESS

When we willingly "open up" and make room for pressure, instead of struggling with or getting pushed around by it, then we massively increase our choices in life.

LIVING YOUR VALUES

Come back to your core values and let them guide you. This could involve going with the pressure, or against the pressure, or another option altogether. You choose!

OBSERVING

Sometimes we feel pressure from others. Sometimes we feel the pressure within ourselves, such as when we feel guilty, or a sense of obligation to exercise or diet. Write down the top 10 things you feel pressured to do (in no particular order).

1. _____
2. _____
3. _____
4. _____
5. _____
6. _____
7. _____
8. _____
9. _____
10. _____

Now, take a moment to observe the thoughts, feelings and sensations that arise within your body, associated with these pressures.

- What kind of guilt trips, judgments, criticisms, threats, "shoulds" and "musts" does your mind say to you?

- What kind of emotions show up? Guilt? Anxiety? Fear? Frustration? Sadness? Impatience?
- What kind of sensations arise in your body? Sweaty hands? Tight chest? Heavy shoulders? Tense forehead? Knotted stomach? Clenched jaws? Tight throat? A sinking feeling?

Please write down what you observe (and if you're not willing to write it, then at least do it in your head).

Pressure thoughts: _____
_____

Pressure feelings: _____
_____

Pressure sensations: _____
_____

WILLINGNESS

Now we would like to take a moment, if you're willing, to open up and make room for your thoughts, feelings and sensations of pressure. Why would you bother to do this? Because it frees you up; it liberates you; it massively expands the choices available to you. The aim of this exercise is to help you to form a new relationship with pressure, that is probably radically different from the one you have had before.

In this new relationship, you will not "give in" to the pressure. Nor will you "rebel" against it. You will not fight it, or suppress it, or try to distract yourself from it. Nor will you get overwhelmed by it, or bogged down in it. And you certainly will not like it, want it or approve of it. Instead, you will "open up" to pressure: become more aware of it, more unhooked from it and more at peace with it. And, as a result, you'll be far more able to choose the life that you care about.

Think about a time you felt pressured to do something. Maybe you felt pressured to diet, or exercise, or look a certain way—or maybe it was something else not even remotely connected with your weight or body. Just take a moment to really connect with that feeling of pressure.

We're going to ask you to think of that pressure as an object, and imagine taking that object out of your body, and placing it about 3 feet in front of you. And then we will ask you to put the object back inside you. Now, before we do so, notice what your mind is saying. Is it protesting that this is silly, or is it being wildly enthusiastic, or is it insisting that this won't work? Or has it perhaps gone silent? Notice that whatever your mind's reaction is—positive, negative or neutral—you can still carry on with the exercise—and we hope that you do!

So, first off, imagine your pressure is an object inside your body, and imagine that you somehow, in some magical way, take that object, lift it out of your body, and place it about 3 feet in front of you. Now take a good look at this object—observe it with great curiosity, as if you're a scientist who has never encountered anything like it before. And then describe it, using the prompts below. (Writing your observations is always best, but again, if you're not willing to write, then at least formulate clear answers inside your head.) When you imagine this pressure as an object:

- How big is it?
- What shape is it?
- What color(s) is it?
- Is it transparent or opaque?
- What temperature is it?
- Are there any hot spots or cold spots within it?
- Is it light, heavy or weightless?
- Is it moving or still?
- If moving, where to and at what speed?
- Is it liquid, solid, gaseous, or more like an "energy field"?
- Is there any vibration, pulsation or sound?
- What is the surface like: rough, smooth, shiny, dull, spiky, gooey, hot, cold, etc.?
- How do you feel about this object? Do you feel repulsed, angry at it, afraid of it, maybe even hatred toward it?

Willingness means opening up and "holding" a feeling we don't necessarily like; holding it softly, gently, kindly. Holding that feeling as if it is a crying baby or a rare, precious butterfly. In other words, we hold these feelings in a mindful, gentle, curious way, rather than in a grit-your-teeth-and-put-up-with-it way. Of course, this doesn't come naturally to us; we don't like feelings of pressure. But learning to hold them gently, and make room for them, is a skill well worth learning.

So, now that you have looked at your "pressure object," we are going to ask you to pick it up, hold it gently, and take it back inside you. Imagine either taking a deep breath in and inhaling the pressure back inside your body, or just picking it up and gently placing it inside you.

Your mind may try to stop you from doing this. It may shout, protest, yell, "I don't want it back. Keep it away." If so, acknowledge that; it's perfectly okay to have those thoughts. Let your mind protest away, and take this object and place it back inside you. Breathe into it and make lots and lots of space for it inside your body.

Once you have done that, push your feet into the floor, straighten your back, and anchor yourself in the present moment. Your aim now is to cultivate a broad awareness: of your body and of the pressure inside it, but also of the world around you. Think of life as being like a stage show: on that stage are all your thoughts and feelings, and everything you can see, hear, touch, taste and smell. This "pressure" is just one aspect of the stage show. Keep a spotlight on the "pressure," but also bring up the lights on the rest of the show. So, open your eyes and ears, and notice what you can see, hear, touch, taste and smell. You might even find it helpful to say something to yourself like: "Here's pressure. I don't like it or want it, but I can make room for it." (Some people find this helpful, some don't; try it out, and if it works for you, use it, and if it doesn't, don't.) Once you've made room for this pressure, the next step is to:

LIVING YOUR VALUES

When we feel pressured, we often do one of two things:

1. We obey the pressure but feel bad about it (angry, resentful, disappointed).
2. We rebel against the pressure—actively fight or resist it, or do the very opposite to prove how strong we are.

In both these cases, we are reacting to the pressure. In response to pressure, you can obey or you can rebel. But there is a third option: you can see and hear the pressure, but choose what you want to do with it. This may involve behavior that looks like obeying (making the healthy choice) or rebelling (making the high-calorie choice), or doing something totally different. The key point is that you are choosing the best behavior for yourself in that moment, rather than merely reacting to pressure. Notice how in the third option you have more choices.

Pressure-free living?

"Pressure-free living" doesn't mean that there is no pressure in your life. There will always be pressures of one form or another. (We imagine that you feel pressure just doing these exercises.) But you can learn to free yourself from the influence of pressure; to choose consciously, deliberately, mindfully to act in line with your values. There's a huge difference between eating green veggies because you consciously choose to nurture your body, and eating green veggies because you feel guilty that you're overweight or because your mind says you *should* lose weight. The former gives you vitality; the latter sucks the life out of you. Similarly, contrast the difference between (a) eating a chocolate mindfully—enjoying it, slowing down and savoring every bite—guided by values of sensuality, having fun, and enhancing pleasure; and (b) wolfing down a box of chocolates to rebel against people who say you should diet.

So, more and more, see if you can make choices based on values, rather than obeying or rebelling against pressure. And when you do make a values-guided choice, learn from it: notice the difference it makes in your life—and, very importantly, congratulate yourself. (If you're anything like us, you'll have to do a hell of a lot of self-congratulation to come anywhere close to equalling your self-criticism.) And when pressure dictates your actions, rather than values . . . then also learn from it: notice the difference it makes in your life, and very importantly, be kind to yourself.

WEEK 4: PRACTICING SELF-COMPASSION

We hope that, after our last exercise, you made contact with the sources of pressure in your life and practiced responding flexibly to that pressure. Just as the weather continually changes, pressure will continually come and go, rise and fall, intensify and diminish. The key is to make room for those feelings of pressure, to create space in order to choose what is consistent with your values.

This week, we are going to explore in greater depth our capacity for self-criticism and self-compassion.

As we have discussed earlier, self-compassion basically means being kind to yourself. It means you recognize and acknowledge that you are in pain and you do something to reduce your suffering, rather than increase it. Self-compassion involves all the O.W.L. skills:

OBSERVING

The first step is to be a curious observer. Notice when and how your inner critic is beating you up. Notice what words it uses to judge and criticize.

WILLINGNESS

Next, make room for all the thoughts and feelings of self-criticism. Take a step back, and give your inner critic plenty of space to scream or shout.

LIVING YOUR VALUES

The last part of self-compassion involves living a particular value: kindness. Instead of being tough on yourself, you treat yourself kindly and gently—using kind thoughts, and kind actions.

USING O.W.L. FOR SELF-COMPASSION

Observing

Your job over the next week is to observe yourself like a curious anthropologist: notice under what circumstances your self-criticism happens. Is it after you've overeaten, or yelled at the kids, or avoided exercise, or failed to follow through on an important goal? And notice what the ritual involves: notice the chants, and rhythms of your mind. Does it repeat a word: "Stupid! Stupid! Stupid!?" Does it express disbelief: "I can't believe I just did that!?" Does it swear: "What a f****** idiot!'? Does it lay a guilt trip on you, dredge up the past, compare you to others? As you spend time observing this self-critic, make some reflections and write them down:

My mind tends to criticize me at the following times,
places, and situations . . .

Next, think of some area of life where you have gone off-track—think about what you did, and see if you can get your inner critic to have a go at you. Then mindfully observe what it does, and describe it below, using our prompts.

- What does your inner critic sound like emotionally (angry, sad, frustrated, anxious, guilty, cold, loathing, disgusted)?

- What is the voice quality (screaming, shrill, shouting, screechy)?
- What is the speed of the voice (fast, slow, normal)?
- Whose voice does it most sound like (your own, one of your parents" voices, someone else)?
- What is the volume of the voice (loud, soft, normal, a whisper)?
- What is the rhythm of the voice (continuous, short bursts, etc.)?

Willingness

As far as we know, there is no way to get rid of your inner critic. We have never met or heard of a human being who doesn't have one. As you embrace and practice the ACT approach, you will probably find that the inner critic goes quiet for periods, but it won't magically disappear. Sooner or later it will return, and it's likely to be especially loud when you're having a difficult time. So let's learn how to live with it in a way that maximizes our wellbeing.

Willingness means that we stop rebelling against the inner critic (debating with it and trying to disprove it with logic, or squashing it with positive affirmations, or pushing it out of our head). It also means that we stop letting it push us around. Instead, we open up and make room for it, and give it plenty of space to have its tantrum. In the meantime, while it's letting off steam, we invest our time and energy in doing something meaningful and life-enhancing.

When you observe your thoughts with curiosity, you're already well on the way to willingness, and the next exercise can help you to really open up.

Imagine your inner critic as an entity, personality, or character of some sort—perhaps like a character from a movie, or a book, or a comic.

- What form does it take? Does it look human or animal, or is it just an abstract shape or color?
- If it has no form, if it is just a formless voice, where in your head does it reside; at the front, at the back, inside your mouth, at the top of your skull?
- Is it male or female or non-specific?
- What is its favorite catchphrase or insult?
- If you gave the critic a name, what would you name it? (For example, one of our clients named his inner critic Nasty Nigel.)
- If you turned it into a cartoon character or movie character what would it look like? (The client mentioned above saw "Nasty Nigel" as a giant purple gorilla. Another client saw his critic as a grumpy old man.)

Now see if you can make room for this character/voice. You might find it helpful to say to yourself, with a sense of humor, "Aha! There you are, inner critic. Have a nice day. Feel free to rant and rave as much as you like." Or you might imagine and talk to it like it's a character in a book or movie: "Aha! Nasty Nigel, I see you've come back to taunt me." Or you might just say to yourself, "Critic time again."

However, if this sort of playful self-talk is not your style, that's no problem. Instead, you might just take a deep breath, and acknowledge the presence of the inner critic without using any words at all—in the same way you might silently nod your head at an acquaintance on the other side of the street.

Basically, you just take a step back and see the critic for what it is—words and pictures inside your head—and let it do what it does. (Tip: many people find a slow, deep breath or two helps this process.) With practice, you can do this very quickly, in the space of a few seconds.

Living your values

The last part of self-compassion involves living a particular value: kindness. You might call it "kindness toward yourself" or "self-care." Now imagine for a moment someone you love without reservation. Bring an image of that person to mind. Once you have this image clear, imagine this person you love so completely was suffering with the doubts and fears that you struggle with under similar circumstances. How would you care for this person? How would you speak to them? What would you say? Write down a few words about how you would ideally like to treat someone you care about, if you knew they were suffering.

Now the big question: are you willing to live these values in your relationship with yourself? If so, what are some kind words you might say to yourself, or some kind things you might do for yourself, in order to develop self-compassion? Write them down.

The benefits of self-compassion

We are not asking you to believe that self-compassion is the best alternative. We are merely encouraging you to give it a try. See if you can be self-compassionate and notice the effects it has. Does it help you live more consciously by your values, or less so? Does it help you achieve more of your goals, or less? Do it as an experiment; play around with it; be curious about the results.

In finishing up, we invite you to use your O.W.L. skills to write a compassionate letter to yourself. The letter should have three elements.

Observing
Notice, with curiosity, what your inner critic is doing. Notice that these criticisms are made up of words—and those words continually come and go. Notice that sometimes the critic is going crazy and screaming wildly, and sometimes it is completely silent.

Willingness
Be willing to let those words come and stay and go in their own good time, as they choose. Let your mind spout all those words about how flawed you are. Make room for the "not good enough" story.

Living your values
Now, from this mental space of curiosity and willingness, deliberately tap into your kindness, warmth and caring, and put self-compassion into play. Write a letter to yourself and think about what you would say to a friend (real or imaginary) in your situation, (or what you would ideally love a good friend to say to you). Try to have a kind understanding of the distress and self-criticism that shows up.

We encourage you to write whatever comes to you. This letter may take about 5 to 15 minutes to write. Note: You cannot do this task incorrectly. It is impossible to fail! Whatever you say is fine. It can be as long or as short as you like—two sentences or two hundred. We invite you to consider finishing it with an expression of support, such as "I'm here for you," or "I'd like to help you out—let me know if there's anything I can do."

This exercise is far more powerful if you actually write the letter, and perhaps mail it to yourself for later. Or you might give the letter to a friend who cares about you and have them mail it to you when you are going through a difficult time. If you are not willing to write the letter, then please at least take the time to compose it in your head.

A COMPASSIONATE LETTER

Dear (insert your name here),

_____

_____

_____

_____

_____

_____

_____

_____

WEEK 5: DEVELOPING MINDFULNESS OF EATING AND DIET

Welcome to Week 5. We hope you're continuing to apply your O.W.L. skills to make choices based on your values rather than letting "pressure" dictate what you do, and to be kind and compassionate to yourself when you screw up or go off-track. And we'd be shocked and stunned (and to be honest, we wouldn't really believe you) if you told us you'd been doing all of this perfectly.

The fact is, we're all imperfect, fallible human beings. We all screw up repeatedly and go off-track, so let's not get hooked by perfectionist ideas and unrealistic expectations. For the whole rest of our life, no matter how many self-help books we read or personal development courses we enroll in, the fact is, we will screw up and go off-track again and again and again and again. And the beautiful thing is, no matter how many times this happens—a million or a billion or a trillion—as soon as we realize what we're doing, we have a choice: we can continue doing what we're doing, or we can use our O.W.L. skills to get back on track.

So even if you spent the whole of the last week overeating, neglecting your values, and avoiding exercise, in this moment, right now, you can get back on track. For example, if your mind's beating you up, you could unhook yourself from the story, and say something kind to yourself such as, "I'm only human, and this stuff is really hard. It's not easy to change old habits." And then you could remind yourself, "I can get back on track any time I choose to. The journey of a thousand miles begins with one step."

Becoming aware of non-hungry eating

We have already discussed the many reasons for non-hungry eating, and so provide just a brief reminder of these below:

- **Habit:** We eat automatically, out of habit. Some event or happening—either inside our body or in the world around us—triggers our desire to eat, and without any self-awareness, we start consuming food.
- **Cravings:** We have a strong temptation or desire for something specific, such as sweets or chips or pizza.
- **Sharing:** We eat to share, socialize, and bond with others.
- **Discomfort:** We eat to comfort ourselves, to improve our mood, or to distract ourselves from unpleasant feelings, such as anxiety, loneliness or boredom.

This week we are going to build our awareness of non-hungry eating so that we can make more values-consistent choices in our eating behavior. You can download two mindfulness exercises from our website, TheWeightEscape.com: the hunger meditation will help you practice recognising cues for true hunger, while the urge surfing meditation will help you to recognize cravings and learn to surf them so that they don't dominate your behavior.

Perhaps one of the best ways to become mindful of what drives your eating is by keeping a mindfulness-based food diary. We have provided you two types of food diaries on the following pages. You choose the one that is most relevant to your particular needs.

Both the diaries ask you to get in touch with your hunger cues. This is perhaps the most important aspect of body wisdom (Chapter 6). But each diary also varies in its emphasis. If you experience a great deal of emotional eating, you might use the Reduce Emotional Eating diary. The most important thing is not the particular food diary you use, but that you practice becoming aware of your hunger cues and when you eat. You might be quite surprised at what you discover. Give it a try!

REDUCE EMOTIONAL EATING: SPOT THE FOOD AND MOOD CYCLES

DATE: _____   MON TUE WED THURS FRI SAT SUN

TIME	FOOD TRIGGERS	FOOD	FEELINGS BEFORE EATING	HUNGRY? (Y/N)	FEELINGS AFTER EATING	WAS EATING THIS FOOD CONSISTENT WITH YOUR VALUES? (CIRCLE ONE)
						Yes Somewhat No
						Yes Somewhat No
						Yes Somewhat No
						Yes Somewhat No
						Yes Somewhat No
						Yes Somewhat No
						Yes Somewhat No
						Yes Somewhat No
						Yes Somewhat No

FOOD TRIGGERS REFER TO THE ASPECTS OF YOUR ENVIRONMENT, IF ANY, THAT TRIGGERED EATING.

WEEKLY HEALTH DIARY

CIRCLE YOUR HUNGER LEVEL WHEN YOU START EATING AND THEN AGAIN WHEN YOU FINISH EATING

DAY/TIME	FOOD OR BEVERAGE	HUNGER SCALE
		1 2 3 4 5 6 7 8 9
		1 2 3 4 5 6 7 8 9
		1 2 3 4 5 6 7 8 9
		1 2 3 4 5 6 7 8 9
		1 2 3 4 5 6 7 8 9
		1 2 3 4 5 6 7 8 9
		1 2 3 4 5 6 7 8 9
		1 2 3 4 5 6 7 8 9
		1 2 3 4 5 6 7 8 9
		1 2 3 4 5 6 7 8 9
		1 2 3 4 5 6 7 8 9
		1 2 3 4 5 6 7 8 9

HUNGER SCALE

1	2	3	4	5	6	7	8	9
Starving, weak		Hunger pangs		Comfortably full		Overfull		So full it hurts

WEEK 6: DEVELOPING AUTHENTIC MOTIVATION TO EXERCISE

This week we are going to talk about an important dimension of your health: physical activity. Let's see if there is a way to align your activity levels more closely with your values.

Has life become too easy?

Technology makes it virtually unnecessary for us to do any physical exercise. We do not have to chop wood to build a fire and generate warmth. Cars release us from walking, escalators release us from climbing stairs, and TV releases us from having to entertain ourselves. Agriculture and supermarkets give us food without us having to hunt or garden. Frozen meals save us the trouble of preparing our meal.

Let's face it; we don't *have* to exercise any more. This means that exercise often requires self-discipline and can feel like work. What's most interesting is that we often don't keep to our exercise plans even though we all know how important exercise is for our health and wellbeing.

BENEFITS OF EXERCISE
- Improves mood (less depression, anxiety and tension)
- Reduces cardiovascular disease
- Improves immune function (for moderate exercise)
- Reduces risk of some cancers
- Reduces risk of Type 2 diabetes
- Improves brain function in older adults; reduces risk of dementia
- Improves quality of sleep
- Helps with weight loss
- Reduces risk of death

OTHER INTERESTING FACTS ABOUT EXERCISE
- Physical activity and a calorie-restricted diet together are more effective for weight loss than calorie restriction alone.
- Physical activity has a positive effect on your body composition, by preserving or increasing lean body mass, while promoting fat loss.
- Increasing exercise generally leads to increase in weight loss (but consult your doctor for suitable level of exercise).

How to increase internal motivation

Research shows that the more people are internally motivated, the more likely they are to stay on an exercise regime. If you feel low motivation to exercise, then you are certainly not alone.

Let's first take a look at the kinds of thoughts that might feel like barriers to exercise and lower your motivation. Remember, the first skill in O.W.L. is observing, so it is important to notice what your mind is telling you about exercise.

THOUGHTS THAT YOUR MIND THROWS AT YOU TO DISCOURAGE YOU FROM EXERCISING

Circle those that hook you, i.e., that you believe sometimes

- Exercise is too much effort
- Exercise requires too much commitment
- I have too many chores to exercise
- Social commitments get in the way of exercise
- I am too stressed to exercise
- I am too sad to exercise
- Nobody encourages me to exercise
- Someone criticizes me for exercising
- I can't exercise after a long day
- I do not have nice places to walk in the neighborhood
- I do not think my neighborhood is safe enough to jog or walk
- I am not the physically active type
- Exercise is for those who do nothing during the day

- Exercise at a gym costs too much
- Gyms are too far away
- I do not know how to exercise properly
- If I exercise, I might hurt myself
- I am too old to exercise
- I am too heavy to exercise
- I feel too shy or embarrassed to exercise
- I have trouble organizing my life to make time for exercise
- I cannot get into an exercise routine
- Work demands too much of my time
- I feel too worn out to exercise
- Exercise is boring
- My family obligations get in the way of exercising
- Other reasons for not exercising (write in your own words)

Now, take a look at those reasons for not exercising. Could you carry one of those reasons with you while you exercise? (Perhaps even put it on a card and carry it with you to the gym.) Do these thoughts have to act as barriers?

If the thought is genuinely pointing to a problem (e.g., your neighborhood is dangerous and you don't want to walk in it), can you problem-solve ways around it (e.g., do a different kind of exercise)?

MOTIVATIONS TO EXERCISE: **IDENTIFY SOME "HEART-FELT" REASONS WHY YOU MIGHT WANT TO EXERCISE**

Now that we have looked at reasons our mind generates for not exercising, let's look at some intrinsic reasons for why people do exercise. Please circle the ones that apply to you:

- Exercise helps me to cope with stress
- Exercise is a good way to clear my thinking
- Exercise helps me to relax
- I feel invigorated after exercising
- Exercise gives me some space to think
- Exercise helps me to prevent health problems
- Exercise helps me to have a healthy body
- Exercise helps me to live longer
- Exercise helps me to have more energy

- Exercise helps me to be attractive
- Exercise gives me the opportunity to spend time with others
- I enjoy the competitive part of exercise
- I love to feel challenged
- I love to exert myself
- Exercise is a good way to have fun
- Exercise is a good way to meet new friends
- Other motives for exercise (write in your own words)

Now that you have looked at motives for exercise, are you ready to consider what you might do to increase your exercise? Can you think of activities that connect to your motives above (e.g., to make exercise fun or social or entertaining)? For example, if you don't want to go to the gym, are there other things you can do?

There are at least two ways to increase your physical activity. First, you can increase the amount of formal exercise that you do—for instance, you can plan to go to the gym three times a week. Second, you can seek to reduce sedentary activity by increasing informal exercise. For example, instead of watching TV for an hour, you can go for a walk and listen to your favorite music or reconnect with nature. Instead of reading a book on the couch, you can exercise while listening to an audio book.

When thinking about physical activity, let yourself be playful and creative. You don't have to do what everybody else is doing or tells you. You can find your own physical activity routine, one that matches your values and interests.

WEEK 7: PULLING EVERYTHING TOGETHER—THE FIVE-STEP PLAN TO CHANGING YOUR LIFE

The final week takes you from values to concrete goals. It shows what you need to do to maximise your chances of achieving your goals.

Steps 1 and 2 of the exercise are to connect your goals to values. As we have argued throughout the book, if you do not know why you are doing something, then you are unlikely to stay committed to it.

Steps 3 and 4 have you generating the benefits and barriers related to the goal. This phase is crucial. It involves keeping the positive (benefits) and the negative (barriers) together. We argued in Chapter 2 that much of our suffering is caused by our attempt to remove the bad parts of life from the good parts. We often can't separate the two.

Step 5 involves making plans. When setting goals, it is not enough to say something like, "I'll try to exercise in the morning." We need to anticipate the barriers that are likely to show up when striving for the goal, and we need to make an if-then plan for what we will do when they arrive. In the above example, an if-then plan might be, "If I don't have much time to exercise, then I will exercise for only 10 minutes instead of 30." Or consider the example where you are seeking to cut down on your calories but are invited out for a meal with your friends. You might say, "If I go out to eat with my friends, then I will eat slowly and mindfully."

Five steps to changing your life

1. Identify guiding values. Values are like guiding stars. You set course by them, but never actually reach them or permanently realize them (e.g., being healthy, mindful, etc.).
2. Set achievable goals that are consistent with your values.
3. Identify benefits. Imagine the most positive outcome of achieving your goals.
4. Identify critical difficulties. Imagine the potential obstacles that might stand in the way of you achieving your goals, be they internal (e.g., self-doubt, anger, etc.) or external.
5. Make commitments.

EXERCISE: **COMMITMENT**

Write down values you want to commit to, opportunities when you can put those values into play, and identify potential difficulties and solutions to them.

I commit to _____ (your goal)

COMMITMENT OPPORTUNITIES

The following are some opportunities for me to put my commitment into play.

Example: If I am at a restaurant, then I will order steamed vegetables instead of garlic bread.

If _____ ,
then I will _____ .

If _____ ,
then I will _____ .

If _____ ,
then I will _____ .

If _____ ,
then I will _____ .

COMMITMENT DIFFICULTIES

If _____
(difficult internal experience, e.g., feelings) shows up, then I will use my observing skills and make room for the experience. If I am unwilling to have the experience, I will pick a goal that is less difficult for me.

If _____
(external difficulty) comes up, then I will _____ .

APPENDIX
NUTRITION GUIDELINES

ESTIMATING ENERGY DENSITY

Low energy density: You can eat satisfying portions of these foods

Medium energy density: Practice portion control

High energy density: Limit portions or substitute food from lower categories

Please note that the estimates in the following tables are based on the USDA website, http://www.ars.usda.gov/. These estimates may vary depending on brand of the foodstuff and the way the food is prepared for eating (e.g., deep fried versus steamed). To estimate exact category of the brand you are eating, divide calories or kilojoules by serving size in grams and use the following table.

CALORIE ENERGY DENSITY	KILOJOULE ENERGY DENSITY	CATEGORY
0–1.5	0–6.3	LOW
1.5–4.0	6.3–16.8	MEDIUM
4.0–9.0	16.8–37.8	HIGH

Example: Calories in a serving of Homestead Seed and Grain Bread = 253. Serving size = 100 grams.

Divide 253 by 100. This gives you 2.53, or a medium category food. Notice that when the serving size is 100, you can just move the decimal place two points to the left to get your energy density. So 253 becomes 2.53.

Warning: Calorie content of the same foodstuff (e.g., basmati rice) can vary significantly depending on the brand and the way it is prepared. The following tables are meant to give you a rough idea of food category, but it is always more accurate to estimate food category by dividing calories (or kilojoules) by serving size as above.

Use the following tables as a first approximation, not as the "ultimate truth." If you add things to the food, then the table will not give accurate numbers. For example, adding cheese sauce to pasta will probably increase the energy density of your dinner. Adding low-fat milk to cereal lowers the average energy density of your breakfast.

LOW ENERGY DENSITY

EAT SATISFYING PORTIONS (ESPECIALLY IF UNDER 4.3)
ENERGY DENSITY (KILOJOULES PER 100G)   0—6.3

BREAKFAST CEREALS

OATMEAL (REGULAR/QUICK/INSTANT OATS) BOILED WITH WATER AND SALT	2.7
BREAKFAST CEREAL BEVERAGE (ALL FLAVORS)	3.4

FRUITS AND VEGETABLES

LETTUCE, ICEBERG, RAW	0.4
CUCUMBER, WITH PEEL, RAW	0.5
CELERY, RAW	0.6
TOMATOES, RED, RAW	0.7
CABBAGE, SAVOY, BOILED, DRAINED WITHOUT SALT	0.9
CAULIFLOWER, BOILED, DRAINED WITHOUT SALT	1.0
MUSHROOMS, WHITE, RAW	1.0
RED OR GREEN PEPPERS	1.0
STRAWBERRIES	1.1
SPINACH, BOILED AND DRAINED WITHOUT SALT	1.2
MELON, CANTELOUPE	1.2
BROCCOLI, BOILED, DRAINED WITHOUT SALT	1.3
CARROTS, RAW OR BOILED, DRAINED WITHOUT SALT	1.3
WATERMELON	1.3
PAPAYA, RAW	1.4
GRAPEFRUIT, RAW (PINK, RED, WHITE)	1.4
ORANGES, VALENCIA	1.5
APRICOTS, RAW	1.7
PEACHES, RAW	1.9
PUMPKIN, BOILED AND DRAINED WITHOUT SALT	1.9
BEETS (CANNED AND DRAINED OR FRESH, PEELED, BOILED AND DRAINED)	2.0
BLUEBERRIES, RAW	2.2
APPLES, RAW WITH SKIN	2.3
MANGOES	2.3
PEARS, RAW	2.4
CHERRIES, RAW	2.5
GREEN PEAS (FROZEN), BOILED AND DRAINED	2.6
GRAPES, RED/GREEN (E.G., THOMPSON SEEDLESS)	2.8
PINEAPPLE	3.0
BANANAS, RAW	3.8
SWEET CORN KERNELS (FROZEN), BOILED AND DRAINED WITHOUT SALT	4.5

DAIRY/EGGS

YOGURT, LOW FAT (<0.5 PERCENT), STRAWBERRY PIECES OR FLAVOURED	3.4
YOGURT, NATURAL, REGULAR FAT (~4 PERCENT)	3.7
YOGURT, REGULAR FAT (~3 PERCENT), STRAWBERRY PIECES OR FLAVORED	4.2
COTTAGE CHEESE	5.3
ICE CREAM, FAT FREE, VANILLA FLAVORED	5.8
EGG, HARD BOILED	5.8
EGG, POACHED	6.3

BREAD AND STAPLES

BULGUR WHEAT (COOKED)	0.8
BUCKWHEAT (COOKED)	0.9
PASTA IN TOMATO SAUCE (CANNED, NO MEAT)	2.3
POTATOES, WHITE, BOILED IN SKIN, FLESH EATEN WITHOUT SALT	2.6
SPLIT PEAS (DRIED), BOILED WITHOUT SALT	2.7
SWEET POTATO, BOILED WITHOUT SKIN	3.2
LENTILS (DRIED), BOILED WITHOUT SALT	3.2
BEANS (CANNED), IN TOMATO SAUCE	3.6
CHINESE RICE STICK NOODLES, BOILED, DRAINED	3.7
INSTANT MASHED POTATO, PREPARED WITH WATER AND MARGARINE	4.0
POTATOES, WHITE, FLESH AND SKIN BAKED	4.2
PEARLED BARLEY, COOKED	4.2
KIDNEY BEANS (CANNED), RINSED WITH TAP WATER	4.2
RICE, WILD, COOKED	4.3
CHICKPEAS (CANNED), DRAINED AND RINSED WITH TAP WATER	4.5
CORNMEAL, WHOLE GRAIN, YELLOW	4.5
MASHED POTATOES, PREPARED WITH MILK AND MARGARINE	4.5
MEAT RAVIOLI	5.7
SPAGHETTI COOKED FROM DRY WITHOUT SALT	5.9
GNOCCHI, BOILED	6.2

COOKED MEAT AND SEAFOOD

TILAPIA, FILLET, BAKED, NO ADDED FAT	4.3
JUMBO SHRIMP, PURCHASED COOKED, FLESH ONLY	4.4
HAM, LEG, LEAN	4.7
BEEF, CORNED, 75 PERCENT TRIMMED	4.8
TUNA (CANNED) IN WATER WITHOUT SALT, DRAINED	5.2
BREAM FILLET, BAKED IN FOIL, NO ADDED FAT	5.9
PINK SALMON (CANNED) IN WATER WITHOUT SALT, DRAINED, FLESH ONLY	6.1

SOUPS

FRENCH ONION (INSTANT PACKET), PREPARED WITH WATER	0.3
MINESTRONE VEGETABLE (INSTANT PACKET), PREPARED WITH WATER	1.1
CHICKEN BROTH (INSTANT PACKET), PREPARED WITH WATER	1.7
PEA AND HAM, WITH VEGETABLES (CANNED)	2.2
MANHATTAN CLAM CHOWDER (CANNED)	2.5
CREAM OF CHICKEN (CANNED)	2.8
MEAT AND CHUNKY VEGETABLE (CANNED)	3.8

MEDIUM ENERGY DENSITY

PRACTICE PORTION CONTROL

ENERGY DENSITY (KILOJOULES PER 100G)   6.3—16.8

BREAKFAST CEREALS

ALL BRAN	13.7
RAISIN BRAN	14.1
WHOLE WHEAT BISCUITS	14.1
SPECIAL K	14.2
NATURAL UNTOASTED MUESLI	14.3
SHREDDED WHEAT	14.4
OAT BRAN (QUAKER)	14.4
PUFFED WHEAT	14.9
COCOA PUFFS	15.2
RICE KRISPIES	15.4
ROLLED OATS (RAW)	15.7
CORNFLAKES	15.8
NUTRIGRAIN	16.0
BRAN FLAKES	16.1
CHEERIOS	16.1

FRUITS AND VEGETABLES

AVOCADOS, RAW, COMMON VARIETIES	8.6

DRIED FRUITS

PRUNES, DRIED, UNCOOKED	8.4
APRICOTS, DRIED, UNCOOKED	8.9
DATES	12.1
APPLES, DRIED, UNCOOKED	12.3
RAISINS	13.3

COOKED MEAT AND SEAFOOD

SNAPPER FLESH, BRUSHED WITH OLIVE OIL, GRILLED OR BARBECUED	6.4
CHICKEN BREAST, LEAN, BAKED	6.4
TURKEY BREAST, LEAN, BAKED	6.5
VEAL, DICED, FULLY TRIMMED, DRY FRIED	6.6
TUNA, YELLOW FIN STEAKS, BRUSHED WITH OLIVE OIL, GRILLED OR BARBECUED	6.7
BEEF STIR-FRY CUTS, FAT FULLY TRIMMED, DRY FRIED	6.8
PORK CHOP, LEAN, BARBECUED	6.8
BEEF FILLET STEAK, SEMI-TRIMMED, GRILLED	7.8
BEEF CASSEROLE CUTS, FAT FULLY TRIMMED, COOKED	7.8
CHICKEN, WHOLE BARBECUED, WITH SKIN	8.1
CHICKEN THIGH, LEAN, ROASTED	8.1
BEEF RIBEYE, SEMI-TRIMMED, GRILLED	8.6
PORK LOIN ROAST, LEAN SEPARABLE FAT, ROASTED WITHOUT OIL OR FAT	8.6
LAMB CHOP, FAT FULLY TRIMMED, GRILLED	8.8
PORK CHOP, ROASTED	9.0
TUNA (CANNED) IN VEGETABLE OIL, WITHOUT SALT	8.9

BREADS AND STAPLES

RICE, WHITE, SHORT, MEDIUM OR LONG GRAINED COOKED	6.7
BASMATI RICE, COOKED (MICROWAVE PACK)	6.7
JASMINE RICE, COOKED (MICROWAVE PACK)	8.4
BREAD, PUMPERNICKEL	8.9
BREAD, RYE	9.7
ENGLISH MUFFIN, WHEAT, TOASTED	9.7
BREAD, WHOLE WHEAT	9.8
BREAD, WHOLE/MIXED GRAIN OR MULTIGRAIN	9.9
BREAD, SOY AND FLAXSEED	10.0
BREAD, WHITE	10.3
HAMBURGER/HOT DOG BUN, PLAIN WHITE	10.7
PITA BREAD, WHITE	10.8
BAGEL (E.G., PLAIN, SESAME, POPPY SEED)	11.0
FRENCH FRIES, OVEN-HEATED	12.0
CROISSANT	15.0

DAIRY/EGGS

ICE CREAM, COOKIES AND CREAM	7.9
CREAM, SOUR, LIGHT (~18 PERCENT FAT)	9.3
CHEESE, HALOUMI	10.5
CHEESE, FETA (SHEEP & COWS MILK)	11.7
CHEESE, CAMEMBERT	12.9
CHEESE, MOZZARELLA	13.1
CHOCOLATE CAKE (WITH ICING)	15.3
CREAM, SOUR, FULL FAT	15.4
CHEESE, BLUE VEIN	15.7
CHEESE, CHEDDAR, REGULAR FAT	16.6
EGG, FRIED	10.4

SNACKS

SCONES, PLAIN	11.7
SNICKERS BAR (HIGH FAT)	12.3
SPONGE CAKE, UN-ICED, PREPARED FROM DRY MIX	13.4
POPCORN, AIR POPPED, NO ADDED OIL/SALT	14.2
GRANOLA/MUESLI BAR, OATS, FRUIT AND NUTS	14.5
RYVITA (ORIGINAL)	14.8
BLUEBERRY MUFFIN, LOW-FAT	15.3
DONUT (PLAIN, SUGARED OR GLAZED)	15.6
CRACKERS, WHOLE WHEAT	16.0
RICE CAKES (PLAIN OR BUCKWHEAT)	16.3

HIGH ENERGY DENSITY

LIMIT PORTIONS, SUBSTITUTE FOODS IN LOWER CATEGORY

ENERGY DENSITY (KILOJOULES PER 100G)   16.8–37.8

BREAKFAST CEREALS

MUESLI, TOASTED	16.8
BELVITA BREAKFAST BISCUITS (OATS)	18.8

BREADS AND STAPLES

TACO SHELLS	19.0

COOKED MEAT AND SEAFOOD

SALAMI, HUNGARIAN	17.3
SALAMI, DANISH	18.0
PORK NECK CHOP, SEPARABLE FAT, ROASTED	20.8
PORK CRACKLING, ROASTED, SALTED	21.3
LAMB CHOP, GRILLED	22.5
BEEF TOPSIDE/SILVERSIDE, SEPARABLE FAT, ROASTED	23.2
BEEF RUMP STEAK, GRILLED	23.2
BACON, MIDDLE RASHER WITH FAT, GRILLED	27.5

DAIRY

CREAM, HEAVY	18.8
CHEESE, PARMESAN, FINELY GRATED	19.5
BUTTER, SALTED/UNSALTED	30.4
GHEE (CLARIFIED BUTTER)	37.0

SNACKS

FRUIT, NUT AND SEED BAR	17.1
OATMEAL COOKIE	19.5
POTATO CHIPS, FLAVORED	20.1
COOKIE, CHOCOLATE CHIP	20.2
PORK RIND SNACK	20.4
CORN CHIPS, PLAIN	20.4
CHIP OR CRISP, SOY	20.7
CORN CHIPS, NACHO CHEESE	20.8
CRACKER, CHEESE FLAVORED	20.9
COOKIE, SHORTBREAD STYLE	21.3
HAZELNUT & CHOCOLATE FLAVORED SPREAD	22.6
MILK CHOCOLATE, WITH ADDED MILK SOLIDS	22.1
PISTACHIO NUTS, RAW	23.9
SEEDS, PUMPKIN, HULLED AND DRIED	24.2
SEEDS, SUNFLOWER	24.7
PEANUTS, DRY-ROASTED WITHOUT SALT	26.6
CASHEW NUTS, OIL-ROASTED WITH SALT	26.6

GI AND ENERGY DENSITY TABLE FOR FRIDGE

BREAKFAST CEREAL

LOW GI	
ALL BRAN	30
TRADITIONAL ROLLED OATS	51
SPECIAL K	54
NATURAL MUESLI	40
MEDIUM GI	
NUTRIGRAIN	66
SHREDDED WHEAT	67
MINI WHEATS	58
QUICK OATS	65
HI GI	
CHEERIOS	74
COCOA PUFFS	77
CORNFLAKES	77
WEETABIX	74

BREAD

LOW GI	
DENSE WHOLEGRAIN	36–53
MULTIGRAIN	43–52
RAISIN BREAD	53
SOURDOUGH WHEAT	54
SOY AND FLAXSEED	36
MEDIUM GI	
PITA, WHITE	57
HAMBURGER BUN	61
CROISSANT	67
HIGH GI	
WHITE	71
BAGEL	72
WHITE TURKISH BREAD	87

VEGETABLES

LOW GI	
RAW CARROTS	16
BOILED CARROTS	41
BROCCOLI	10
CABBAGE	10
CAULIFLOWER	15
TOMATOES	15
MEDIUM GI	
BEET	64
HIGH GI	
PUMPKIN	75
PARSNIPS	97
INSTANT MASHED POTATO	86

STAPLES

LOW GI	
NEW POTATOES	54
SPAGHETTI	32
WHEAT PASTA	54
MEAT RAVIOLI	39
RICE NOODLES (FRESH)	40
BROWN RICE	50
WHEAT TORTILLA	30
MEDIUM GI	
BASMATI RICE	58
BAKED POTATO	60
COUSCOUS	61
GNOCCHI	68
TACO SHELLS	68
HIGH GI	
FRENCH FRIES	75
SHORT GRAIN WHITE RICE	83
MASHED POTATOES	73
INSTANT WHITE RICE	87

ENERGY DENSITY

0–6.3	LOW
6.3–16.8	MEDIUM
16.8–37.8	HIGH

FRUITS

LOW GI	
STRAWBERRIES	40
ORANGES	40
KIWI FRUIT	47
CHERRIES	22
GRAPES	43
APPLES	34
PEARS	41
MEDIUM GI	
PINEAPPLE	66
BANANAS	58
MANGO	60
FIGS	61
PAPAYA	60
HIGH GI	
WATERMELON	80
DATES	103

DAIRY

LOW GI	
SOY MILK	44
SKIM MILK	32
WHOLE MILK	31
SWEETENED YOGURT	33
CUSTARD	35
LOW-FAT ICE-CREAM	27–48
MEDIUM GI	
ICE CREAM	62

LEGUMES (BEANS)

LOW GI	
CHICKPEAS	42
LENTILS (GREEN)	30
KIDNEY BEANS (CANNED)	52
BUTTER BEANS	36
BAKED BEANS IN TOMATO SAUCE	49

SNACKS AND SWEET FOOD

LOW GI	
SNICKERS BAR (HIGH FAT)	41
MILK CHOCOLATE	42
CORN CHIPS	42
NUT AND SEED MUESLI BAR	49
PEANUTS	13
NUTS AND RAISINS	21
MEDIUM GI	
BLUEBERRY MUFFIN	59
RYVITA	63
HONEY	58
HIGH GI	
SCONES	92
DONUTS	76
RICE CAKES	87
WATER CRACKERS	78
PRETZELS	83

PORTION SIZES

These illustrations give a rough guide to correct portion sizes for different types of food.

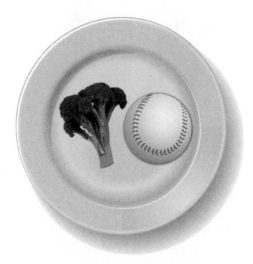

VEGETABLES AND FRUIT
Vegetables: 1 baseball = 1 cup broccoli, beans, raw leafy greens
Fruit: 1 baseball = ½ cup sliced fruit, 1 small apple, 1 medium orange

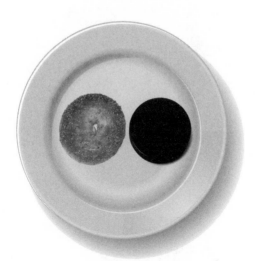

CARBOHYDRATES
1 hockey puck = ½ bagel, ½ cup pasta or dried cereal,
1 slice whole-grain bread, ½ medium potato

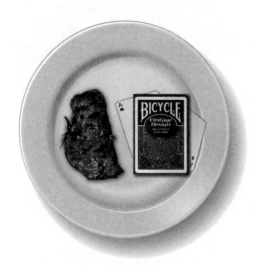

PROTEINS
1 deck of cards = 85 grams of fish;
⅔ deck of cards = 55–70 grams of meat

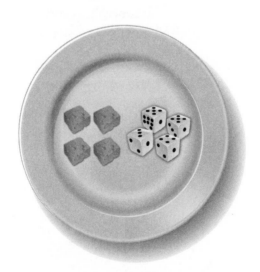

CHEESE
4 dice or about 40–55 grams

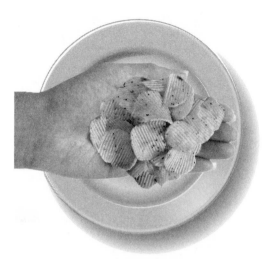

CHIPS AND NUTS
1 small handful

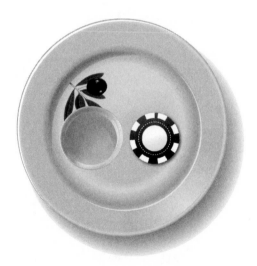

FAT
1 poker chip = 1 teaspoon oil or margarine,
or about 1.5 teaspoons of peanut butter

NOTES

INTRODUCTION

4. "ACT is best known for . . .": Lillis, J., S. C. Hayes, K. Bunting & A. Masuda, "Teaching acceptance and mindfulness to improve the lives of the obese: a preliminary test of a theoretical model," *Annals of Behavioral Medicine,* 2009, in press; Tapper, K., C. Shaw, J. Ilsley, A. Hill, F. Bond & L. Moor, "Exploratory randomised controlled trial of a mindfulness-based weight loss intervention for women," *Appetite,* 2009, vol. 52, pp. 396–404; Weineland, S., D. Arvidsson, T. Kakoulidis & J. Dahl, "Acceptance and commitment therapy for bariatric surgery patients, a pilot RCT," *Obesity Research and Clinical Practice,* 2012, vol. 6, pp. E21–E30; Neimeier, H., T. Leahey, K. Reed, R. Brown & R. Wing, "An acceptance-based behavioral intervention for weight loss: a pilot study," *Behavior Therapy,* 2012, vol. 43, pp. 427–35; Bond, F. W. & D. Bunce, "Mediators of change in emotion-focused and problem-focused worksite stress management interventions," *Journal of Occupational Health Psychology,* 2000, vol. 5, no. 1, pp. 156–63; Juarascio, A., E. Forman & J. Herbert, "Acceptance and commitment therapy versus cognitive therapy for the treatment of co-morbid eating pathology," *Behavior Modification,* 2010, vol. 34, pp. 175–90; Butryn, M., E. Forman, I. Hoffman, J. Shaw & A. Juarascio, "A pilot study of acceptance and commitment therapy for promotion of physical activity," *Journal of Physical Activity and Health,* 2011, vol. 8, pp. 516–22; Goodwin, C., E. Forman, J. Herbert, M. Butryn & G. Ledley, "A pilot study examining the initial effectiveness of a brief acceptance-based behavior therapy for modifying diet and physical activity among cardiac patients," *Behavior Modification,* 2012, vol. 36, pp. 199–217; Pearson, A., V. Follette & S. C. Hayes, "A pilot study of acceptance and commitment therapy as a workshop intervention for body dissatisfaction and disordered eating attitudes," *Cognitive and Behavioral Practice,* 2012, vol. 19, pp. 181–97; Gifford, E. V., B. S. Kohlenberg, S. C. Hayes, D. O. Antonuccio, M. M. Piasecki, M. L. Rasmussen-Hall & K. M. Palm, "Acceptance theory-based treatment for smoking cessation: an initial trial of acceptance and commitment therapy," *Behavior Therapy,* 2004, vol. 35, pp. 689–706; Gregg, J. A., G. M. Callaghan, S. C. Hayes & J. L. Glenn-Lawson, "Improving diabetes self-management

through acceptance, mindfulness, and values: a randomized controlled trial," *Journal of Consulting and Clinical Psychology*, 2007, vol. 75, no. 2, pp. 336–43.

7. "Fortunately, scientific research indicates . . .": Sacks, F., G. Bray, V. Carey, S. Smith, D. Ryan, S. Anton, K. McManus, C. Champagne, L. Bishop, N. Laranjo *et al.*, "Comparison of weight-loss diets with different compositions of fat, protein, and carbohydrates," *New England Journal of Medicine*, 2009, vol. 360, pp. 859–73; Franz, M. J., J. J. VanWormer, A. L. Crain, J. L. Boucher, T. Histon, W. Caplan, J. D. Bowman & N. P. Pronk, "Weight-loss outcomes: a systematic review and meta-analysis of weight-loss clinical trials with a minimum 1-year follow-up," *Journal of the American Dietetic Association*, 2007, vol. 107, no. 10, pp. 1755–67; Jeffery, R. W., A. Drewnowski, L. H. Epstein, A. J. Stunkard, G. T. Wilson, R. R. Wing & D. R. Hill, "Long-term maintenance of weight loss: current status," *Health Psychology*, 2000, vol. 19, pp. 5–16; Knowler, W. C., E. Barrett-Connor, S. E. Fowler, J. M. Lachin, E. A. Walker & D. M. Nathan (Diabetes Prevention Research Group), "Reduction in the incidence of type 2 diabetes with lifestyle intervention or metformin," *New England Journal of Medicine*, 2002, vol. 346, pp. 393–403; Look AHEAD Research Group & R. R. Wing, "Long term effects of a lifestyle intervention on weight and cardiovascular risk factors in individuals with type 2 diabetes: four year results of the Look AHEAD trial," *Archives of Internal Medicine*, 2010, vol. 170, pp. 1566–75.

PART 1: BREAKING FREE
CHAPTER 1: IDENTIFYING YOUR VALUES AND GOALS

20. "Research suggests that . . .": Kasser, T., *The High Price of Materialism*, MIT Press, Cambridge, Massachusetts, 2002.

20. "People who succeed . . .": Niemiec, C. P., R. M. Ryan & E. L. Deci, "The path taken: consequences of attaining intrinsic and extrinsic aspirations in post-college life," *Journal of Research in Personality*, 2009, vol. 73, pp. 291–306.

22. "Well, amazingly, research shows . . .": Crocker, J. & D. Mischkowski, "Why does writing about important values reduce defensiveness? Self-affirmation and the role of positive other-directed feelings," *Psychological Science*, 2008, vol. 19, pp. 740–47; Cohen, G. L., J. Garcia, N. Apfel & A. Master, "Reducing the racial achievement gap: a social-psychological intervention," *Science*, 2006, vol. 313, pp. 1307–10; Creswell, J. D., W. T. Welch, S. E. Taylor, D. K. Sherman, T. L. Gruenewald & T. Mann, "Affirmation of personal values buffers neuroendocrine and psychological stress responses," *Psychological Science*, 2005, no. 16, pp. 846–51; Thomas, S., B. Bushman, B. Castro & A. Reijntjes, "Arousing 'gentle passions' in young adolescents: sustained experimental effects of value affirmations on prosocial feelings and behaviors," *Developmental Psychology*, 2012, vol. 48, pp. 103–10; Logel, C. & G. Cohen, "The role of the self in physical health: testing the effect of a values-affirmation intervention on weight loss," *Psychological Science*, 2012, vol. 23, pp. 53–55.

30. "Regular aerobic exercise . . .": Smith, P., J. Blumenthal, B. Hoffman, H. Cooper, T. Strauman, K. Welsh-Bohmer, J. Browndyke & A. Sherwood, "Aerobic exercise and neurocognitive performance: a meta-analytic review of randomized controlled trials," *Psychosomatic Medicine*, 2010, vol. 72, pp. 239–52; Guiney, H. & L. Machado, "Benefits of regular aerobic exercise for executive functioning in healthy populations," *Psychonomic Bulletin & Review*, 2012, vol. 20, no. 1, pp. 73–86.

30. "Increased consumption . . .": Letenneur, L., C. Proust-Lima, A. Gouge, J. Dartigues & P. Barberger-Gateau, "Flavonoid intake and cognitive decline over a 10-year period," *American Journal of Epidemiology*, 2007, vol. 165, pp. 1364–71.

30. "Low to moderate . . .": Puetz, T. W., P. J. O'Connor & R. K. Dishman, "Effects of chronic exercise on feelings of energy and fatigue: a quantitative synthesis," *Psychological Bulletin*, 2006, vol. 132, pp. 866–76; Puetz, T. W., S. S. Flowers & P. J. O'Connor, "A randomized controlled trial of the effect of aerobic exercise training on feelings of energy and fatigue in sedentary young adults with persistent fatigue," *Psychotherapy and Psychosomatics*, 2008, vol. 77, pp. 167–74.

30. "Exercise can be . . .": Garber, C., B. Blissmer, M. Deschenes, B. Franklin, M. Lamonte, D. Neiman & D. Swain, "Quantity and quality of exercise for developing and maintaining cardiorespiratory, musculoskeletal, and neuromotor fitness in apparently healthy adults: guidance for prescribing exercise: position statement," *Medicine and Science in Sports and Exercise*, 2011, pp. 1334–59.

30. "It also improves . . .": Singh, N., K. Clements & M. Fiatarone, "Sleep, sleep deprivation, and daytime activities: a randomized controlled trial of the effect of exercise on sleep," *Sleep*, 1997, vol. 20, pp. 95–101.

30. "If you're overweight . . .": Jenkinson, C., M. Doherty, A. Avery, A. Read, M. Taylor & T. Sach, "Effects of dietary intervention and quadriceps strengthening exercises on pain and function in overweight people with knee pain: randomised controlled trial," *British Medical Journal*, 2009, vol. 339, p. 3170; Christensen, R., E. M. Bartels, A. Astrup & H. Bliddal, "Effect of weight reduction in obese patients diagnosed with knee osteoarthritis: a systematic review and meta-analysis," *Annals of Rheumatic Diseases*, 2007, vol. 66, pp. 433–39; Villareal, D., S. Chode, N. Parimi, D. Sinacore, T. Hilton, R. Villareal, N. Napoli, C. Qualls & K. Shah, "Weight loss, exercise, or both and physical function in obese older adults," *New England Journal of Medicine*, 2011, vol. 364, pp. 1218–29.

30. "Exercise reduces the . . .": Garber, C., B. Blissmer, M. Deschenes, B. Franklin, M. Lamonte, D. Neiman & D. Swain, "Quantity and quality of exercise for developing and maintaining cardiorespiratory, musculoskeletal, and neuromotor fitness in apparently healthy adults: guidance for prescribing exercise: position statement," *Medicine and Science in Sports and Exercise*, 2011, pp. 1334–59.

30. "It lowers your . . .": Garber, C., B. Blissmer, M. Deschenes, B. Franklin, M. Lamonte, D. Neiman & D. Swain, "Quantity and quality of exercise for developing and maintaining cardiorespiratory, musculoskeletal, and neuromotor fitness in apparently healthy adults: guidance for prescribing exercise: position statement," *Medicine and Science in Sports and Exercise*, 2011, pp. 1334–59.

30. "Fitness enthusiasts . . .": Nieman, D., "Is infection risk linked to exercise workload?," *Medicine and Science in Sports and Exercise*, 2000, vol. 32, pp. s406–s411.

30. "About 40 minutes . . .": Nieman, D., S. Nehlsen, M. Balk-Laamberton, H. Yang, D. Chritton & K. Arabatzis, "The effects of moderate exercise training on natural killer cells and acute upper respiratory tract infections," *International Journal of Sports Medicine*, 1990, vol. 11, pp. 467–73.

30. "Engaging in moderate . . .": Matthews, C., I. Ochene, M. Freedson, J. Rosal, J. Herbert & P. Merriam, "Physical activity and risk of upper-respiratory tract infection," *Medicine and Science in Sports and Exercise*, 2000, vol. 32, p. s292.

30. "If you're overweight . . .": Aucott, L., H. Rothnie, L. McIntyre, M. Thapa, C. Wameru & D. Gray, "Long-term weight loss from lifestyle intervention benefits blood pressure: a systematic review," *Hypertension*, 2009, pp. 756–62; Galani, C. & H. Schneider, "Prevention and treatment of obesity with lifestyle interventions: review and meta-analysis," *International Journal of Public Health*, 2009, pp. 348–59.

31. "Importantly, modest weight . . .": Uusitupa, M., M. Peltonen, J. Lindstrom, A. Aunola, P. Ilanne-Parikka & S. Keinanen, "Ten-year mortality and cardiovascular morbidity in the Finnish Diabetes Prevention Study—secondary analysis of the randomized trial," *Plos One*, 2009, vol. 4, p. 5656.

31. "That will reduce . . .": Kaur, C. & H. C. Kapoor, "Antioxidants in fruits and vegetables—the millennium's health," *International Journal of Food Science and Technology*, 2001, vol. 36, pp. 703–25; He, F., C. Nowson & G. MacGregor, "Increased consumption of fruit and vegetables is related to a reduced risk of coronary heart disease: meta-analysis of cohort studies," *Journal of Hypertension*, 2007, vol. 21, pp. 717–28.

31. "Exercise reduces stress . . .": Tsatsoulis, A. & S. Fountoulakis, "The protective role of exercise on stress system dysregulation and comorbidities," *Annals of New York Acadamy of Sciences*, 2006, vol. 1083, pp. 196–213.

31. "Research also suggests . . .": Maher, J., S. Doerksen, S. Elavsky, A. Hyde & A. Pincus, "A daily analysis of physical activity and satisfaction with life in emerging adults," *Health Psychology*, 2012, vol. 32, no. 6, pp. 647–56.

31. "If you're overweight, even . . .": Blain, B., J. Rodman, J. Newman, "Weight loss treatment and psychological well-being: a review and meta-analysis," *Journal of Health Psychology*, 2007, vol. 12, pp. 68–82.

31. "The wellbeing benefit . . .": Blanchflower, D. G., A. J. Oswald & S. Stewart-Brown, "Is psychological well-being linked to the consumption of fruit and vegetables?," in *Working Paper Series (National Bureau of Economic Research)*, no. 18469, October 2012.

31. "Self-control or willpower . . .": Gailliot, M. T., R. F. Baumeister, C. N. DeWall, J. K. Maner, E. A. Plant, D. M. Tice, L. E. Brewer & B. J. Schmeichel, "Self-control relies on glucose as a limited energy source: willpower is more than a metaphor," *Journal of Personality and Social Psychology*, 2007, vol. 92, pp. 325–36.

31. "Such people engage . . .": Oaten, M. & K. Change, "Longitudinal gains in self-regulation from regular physical exercise," *British Journal of Health Psychology*, 2006, vol. 11, pp. 717–33.

32. "Just about any . . .": Lautenschlager, N. T., K. L. Cox, L. Flicker, J. K. Foster, F. M. van Bockxmeer, J. Xiao, K. R. Greenop & O. P. Almeida, "Effect of physical activity on cognitive function in older adults at risk for Alzheimer disease," *Journal of the American Medical Association*, 2008, vol. 300, pp. 1027–37; Buchman, A. S., P. A. Boyle, L. Yu, R. C. Shah, R. S. Wilson & D. A. Bennett, "Total daily physical activity and the risk of AD and cognitive decline in older adults," *Neurology*, 2012, vol. 78, pp. 1323–29.

32. "In addition to . . .": Sundell, J., "Resistance training is an effective tool against metabolic frailty syndromes," *Advances in Preventitive Medicine*, 2011, pp. 1–7.

32. "Aerobic exercise, meanwhile, offsets . . .": Haaland, D., T. Sabljic, D. Baribeau, I. Mukovozov & L. Hart, "Is regular exercise a friend or foe of the aging immune system? A systematic review," *Clinical Journal of Sports Medicine*, vol. 18, pp. 539–48.

32. "Note how the thigh . . .": Wroblewski, A. P., Amati, F., M. Smiley, B. Goodpaster & V. Wright. "Chronic exercise preserves lean muscle mass in masters athletes," *The Physician and Sportsmedicine*, 2011, vol. 39, no. 3, pp. 172–8.

34. "Increased intake of fruit . . .": Kaur, C. & H. Kapoor, "Antioxidants in fruits and vegetables—the millennium's health," *International Journal of Food Science and Technology*, 2001, vol. 36, pp. 703–25.

34. "Increased vegetable intake . . .": Letenneur, L., C. Proust-Lima, A. Gouge, J. Dartigues & P. Barberger-Gateau, "Flavonoid intake and cognitive decline over a 10-year period," *American Journal of Epidemiology*, 2007, vol. 165, pp. 1364–71; Kang, J., A. Ascherio & F. Grodstein, "Fruit and vegetable consumption and cognitive decline in aging women," *Annals of Neurology*, 2005, vol. 57, pp. 713–20.

34. "For example, being . . .": Profenno, L., A. Porsteinsson & S. Faraone, "Meta-analysis of Alzheimer's disease risk with obesity, diabetes, and related disorders," *Biological Psychiatry*, 2010, vol. 67, pp. 505–12.

34. "The more unhealthy . . .": Sabia, S., H. Nabi, M. Kivimaki, M. J. Shipley, M. G. Marmot & A. Singh-Manoux, "Health behaviors from early to late midlife as predictors of cognitive function: the Whitehall II Study," *American Journal of Epidemiology*, 2009, vol. 170, pp. 428–37.

34. "This is because . . .": Mendez, J. & A. Keys, "Density and composition of mammalian muscle," Metabolism, 1960, vol. 9, pp 184–188.

CHAPTER 2: RECOVERING YOUR STRENGTH

41. "Community surveys reveal . . .": Kessler, R. C., O. Demier, R. G. Frank, M. Olfson, H. A. Pincus, E. E. Walters, P. Wang, K. B. Wells & A. M. Zaslavsky, "Prevalence and treatment of mental disorders, 1990 to 2003," *New England Journal of Medicine*, 2005, vol. 352, no. 24, pp. 2515–23; Kessler, R. C., K. A. McGonagle, S. Zhao, C. B. Nelson, M. Hughes, S. Eshleman, H. U. Wittchen & K. S. Kendler, "Lifetime and 12-month prevalence of DSM-III–R psychiatric disorders in the United States: results from the National Comorbidity Survey," *Archives of General Psychiatry*, 1994, vol. 51, no. 1, pp. 8–19.

46. "Yet there's no evidence whatsoever . . .": Myers, D. G., *The Pursuit of Happiness: Who Is Happy and Why*, William Morrow, New York, 1992.

CHAPTER 3: FINDING YOUR TIPPING POINT

55. "A tipping point is . . .": Gladwell, M., *The Tipping Point: How Little Things Can Make a Big Difference*, Back Bay Books, New York, 2002, p. 12.

CHAPTER 4: ESCAPING THE CAGE

69. "They experience reductions . . .": Price, D., G. Finniss & F. Benedetti, "A comprehensive review of the placebo effect: recent advances and current thought," *Annual Review of Psychology*, 2008, vol. 59, pp. 565–90.

69. "Research suggests that if people . . .": Kierein, N. & M. Gold, "Pygmalion in work organizations: a meta-analysis," *Journal of Organizational Behavior*, 2000, vol. 21, pp. 913–28.

72. "Our society has . . .": Myers, D. G., *The Pursuit of Happiness: Who Is Happy and Why*, William Morrow, New York, 1992.

72. "This is what psychologists . . .": Vartanian, L. & S. Novak, "Internalized societal attitudes moderate the impact of weight stigma on avoidance of exercise," *Obesity*, 2011, vol. 19, pp. 757–62.

79. "When our thoughts dominate . . .": Hayes, S. C., K. Strosahl & K. G. Wilson. *Acceptance and Commitment Therapy The Process and Practice of Mindful Change* (Second ed.), The Guilford Press, New York, 2011.

CHAPTER 5: HARNESSING THE POWER OF FLEXIBILITY

90. "People who follow rigid . . .": Westenhoefer, J., A. Stunkard & V. Pudel, "Validation of the flexible and rigid control dimensions of dietary restraint," *International Journal of Eating Disorders*, vol. 26, pp. 53–64; Westenhoefer, J., B. Flack, A. Stellfeldt & S. Fintelmann, "Behavioral correlates of successful weight reduction over 3 years: results from the Lean Habits Study," *International Journal of Obesity*, 2004, vol. 28, pp. 334–35.

101. "The key is to practice . . .": B.J. Rolls, L.S. Roe & J.S. Meengs (2006), "Reductions in portion size and energy density of foods are additive and lead to sustained decreases in energy intake," *American Journal of Clinical Nutrition* 83(1): 11–17.

101. "Foods with a high energy . . .": Rolls, B. J., E. M. Bell, V. H. Castellanos, M. Chow, C. L. Pelkman & M. K. Thorwart: "Energy density but not fat content of foods affected energy intake in lean and obese women," *American Journal of Clinical Nutrition*, 1999, vol. 69, pp. 863–71; Bell, E., V. Castellanos, C. Pelkman, M. Thorwart & B. Rolls, "Energy density of foods affects energy intake in normal-weight women," *American Journal of Clinical Nutrition*, 1998, vol. 67, pp. 412–20; Ledikwe, J. H., H. Blanck, L. Khan, M. Serdula, J. Seymour, B. Tohill & B. Rolls, "Dietary energy density is associated with energy intake and weight status in US adults," *American Journal of Clinical Nutrition*, 2006, vol. 83, pp. 1362–68.

101. "The amazing thing is . . .": Blatt, A., L. Roe & B. Rolls, "Hidden vegetables: an effective strategy to reduce energy intake and increase vegetable intake in adults," *American Journal of Clinical Nutrition*, 2011, vol. 93, pp. 756–63.

101. "If you're interested . . .": Rolls, B., *The Ultimate Volumetrics Diet: Smart, Simple, Science-based Strategies for Losing Weight and Keeping It Off*, HarperCollins, New York, 2013.

102. "Lower-GI diets are . . .": Sacks, F., G. Bray, V. Carey, S. Smith, D. Ryan, S. Anton, K. McManus, C. Champagne, L. Bishop, N. Laranjo *et al.*, "Comparison of weight-loss diets with different compositions of fat, protein, and carbohydrates," *New England Journal of Medicine*, 2009, vol. 360, pp. 859–73; Look AHEAD Research Group & R. R. Wing, "Long term effects of a lifestyle intervention on weight and cardiovascular risk factors in individuals with type 2 diabetes: four year results of the Look AHEAD trial," *Archives of Internal Medicine*, 2010, vol. 170, pp. 1566–75; Rizkalla, S. W., F. Bellisle & G. Slama, "Health benefits of low glycaemic index foods, such as pulses, in diabetic patients and healthy individuals," *The British Journal of Nutrition*, 2002, vol. 88, pp. 255–62.

103. "Something with a high . . .": Fuhrman, J., *Eat to Live: The Amazing Nutrient-rich Program for Fast and Sustained Weight Loss*, revised ed., Little, Brown, London, 2012.

103. "Increasing the nutritional . . .": Fuhrman, J., *Eat to Live: The Amazing Nutrient-rich Program for Fast and Sustained Weight Loss*, revised ed., Little, Brown, London, 2012; Liu, R., "Health benefits of fruit and vegetables are from additive and synergistic combinations of phytochemicals," *American Journal of Clinical Nutrition*, 2003, vol. 78, pp. 517–20; van Duyn, M. A. & E. Pivonka, "Overview of the health benefits of fruit and vegetable consumption for the dietetics professional: selected literature," *Journal of the American Dietetic Association*, 2000, vol. 100, pp. 1511–21; Kaur, C. & H. Kapoor, "Antioxidants in fruits and vegetables—the millennium's health," *International Journal of Food Science and Technology*, 2001, vol. 36, pp. 703–25.

103. "One interesting study . . .": Fuhrman, J., B. Sarter, B. Glaser & S. Acolella, "Changing perceptions of hunger on a high nutrient density diet," *Nutrition Journal*, 2010, vol. 9, pp. 1–13.

103. "Regular consumption of whole . . .": Liu, R., "Health benefits of fruit and vegetables are from additive and synergistic combinations of phytochemicals," *American Journal of Clinical Nutrition*, 2003, vol. 78, pp. 517–20.

104. "Unfortunately, after years . . .": Liu, R., "Health benefits of fruit and vegetables are from additive and synergistic combinations of phytochemicals," *American Journal of Clinical Nutrition*, 2003, vol. 78, pp. 517–20; Jacob, R. G., M. Gross M & L. Tapsell, "Food synergy: an operational concept for understanding nutrition," *American Journal of Clinical Nutrition*, 2009, vol. 89, pp. 1s–6s.

104. "Or to take another . . .": Liu, R., "Health benefits of fruit and vegetables are from additive and synergistic combinations of phytochemicals," *American Journal of Clinical Nutrition*, 2003, vol. 78, pp. 517–20.

104. "It turns out these . . .": Heneman, K. & S. Zidenberg-Cherr, Nutrition and Health Info-sheet for Health Professionals, UC Cooperative Extension Center for Health and Nutrition Research, Department of Nutrition, University of California, Davis, California, 2008.

PART 2: BUILDING A NEW LIFE
CHAPTER 7: DEVELOPING THE MINDFULNESS HABIT

130. "Habits begin with . . .": Duhigg, C., *The Power of Habit: Why We Do What We Do and How to Change*, Random House, New York, 2012.

130. "If we do that often . . .": Duhigg, C., *The Power of Habit: Why We Do What We Do and How to Change*, Random House, New York, 2012.

130. "The brain's pleasure . . .": Duhigg, C., *The Power of Habit: Why We Do What We Do and How to Change*, Random House, New York, 2012.

131. "But then, when we . . .": Duhigg, C., *The Power of Habit: Why We Do What We Do and How to Change*, Random House, New York, 2012.

132. "It enables us to shift. . .": Segerstrom, S. C., J. K. Hardy, D. R. Evans & N. F. Windters, 'Pause and plan': self-regulation and the heart," in G. Gendolla & R. Wright (eds), *Motivational Perspectives on Cardiovascular Response: Mechanisms and Applications*, American Psychological Association, Washington, DC, 2011, pp. 181–98.

132. "We now know that . . .": Davis, D. & J. Hayes, "What are the benefits of mindfulness?

A practice review of psychotherapy-related research," *Psychotherapy*, 2011, vol. 48, pp. 198–208.

137. "Deep, slow breathing . . .": Varvogli, L. & C. Darviri, "Stress management techniques: evidence-based procedures that reduce stress and promote health," *Health Science Journal*, 2011, vol. 5, pp. 74–89; Ravinder, J., J. Edry, V. Barnes & V. Jerath, "Physiology of long pranayamic breathing: neural respiratory elements may provide a mechanism that explains how slow deep breathing shifts the autonomic nervous system," *Medical Hypotheses*, 2006, vol. 67, pp. 556–571.

CHAPTER 8: MAKING HARD CHOICES EASIER

147. "The more of these tough . . .": Muraven, M., & R. F. Baumeister. "Self-regulation and depletion of limited resources: does self-control resemble a muscle?," *Psychological Bulletin, 2000, vol. 126*, no. 2, pp. 247–59.

149. "We'll tend to eat a much . . .": Wansink, B. & P. Chandon, "Can 'low-fat' nutrition labels lead to obesity?," *Journal of Marketing Research*, 2006, vol. 18, pp. 605–17.

150. "We'll tend to believe . . .": Wansink, B., K. Ittersum & J. Painter, "How diet and health labels influence taste and satiation," *Journal of Food Science*, 2004, vol. 69, pp. 340–46.

150. "We tend to eat more old . . .": Wansink, B. & J. Kim, "Bad popcorn in big buckets: portion size can influence intake as much as taste," *Journal of Nutrition Education and Behavior*, 2005, vol. 37, pp. 242–45.

150. "We'll eat 69 percent . . .": Kahn, B. & B. Wansink, "The influence of assortment structure on perceived variety and consumption quantities," *Journal of Consumer Research*, 2004, vol. 30, pp. 519–33.

150. "The more people we have . . .": Vartanian, L., C. Herman & B. Wansink, "Are we aware of the external factors that influence our food intake?," *Health Psychology*, 2008, vol. 27, pp. 533–38; de Castro, J. & M. Brewer, "The amount eaten in meals by humans is a function of the number of people present," *Physiology and Behavior*, 1991, vol. 51, no. 1, pp. 121–25.

150. "If our eating companions . . .": McFerran, B., D. W. Dahl, G. J. Fitzsimons & A. C. Morales, "I'll have what she's having: effects of social influence and body type on food choices of others," *Journal of Consumer Research*, 2010, vol. 36, pp. 915–29.

150. "If we have a large meal . . .": Wansink, B. & P. Chandon, "Meal size, not body size, explains errors in estimating the calorie content of meals," *Annals of Internal Medicine*, 2006, vol. 145, pp. 326–32.

151. "Believe it or not . . .": Wansink, B. & J. Sobel, "Mindless eating: the 200 daily food decisions we overlook," *Environment and Behavior*, 2007, vol. 39, pp. 106–23.

151. "If you underestimated . . .": Wansink, B., B. Payne & J. North, "Fine as North Dakota wine: sensory expectations and the intake of companion foods," *Physiology and Behavior*, 2007, vol. 90, pp. 712–16.

151. "Most people are also . . .": Vartanian, L., C. Herman & B. Wansink, "Are we aware of the external factors that influence our food intake?," *Health Psychology*, 2008, vol. 27, pp. 533–38; Wansink, B. & J. Sobel, "Mindless eating: the 200 daily food decisions we

overlook," *Environment and Behavior*, 2007, vol. 39, pp. 106–23; Wansink, B., *Mindless Eating: Why We Eat More Than We Think*, Bantam Books, New York, 2006.

151. "The good news is . . .": Wansink, B., *Mindless Eating: Why We Eat More Than We Think*, Bantam Books, New York, 2006.

151. "Brian Wansink, a renowned . . .": Wansink, B., J. Painter & J. North, "Bottomless bowls: why visual cues of portion size influence intake," *Obesity*, 2004, vol. 13, pp. 93–100.

152. "And right there is . . .": Wansink, B., *Mindless Eating: Why We Eat More Than We Think*, Bantam Books, New York, 2006; Wansink, B. & C. S. Wansink, "The largest Last Supper: depictions of food portions and plate size increased over the millennium," *International Journal of Obesity*, 2010, vol. 34, pp. 943–44; Wansink, B. & C. R. Payne, "The joy of cooking too much: 70 years of calorie increases in classic recipes," *Annals of Internal Medicine*, 2009, vol. 150, no. 4, pp. 291–92.

152. "By 2006, the average . . .": Wansink, B. & C. R. Payne, "The joy of cooking too much: 70 years of calorie increases in classic recipes," *Annals of Internal Medicine*, 2009, vol. 150, no. 4, pp. 291–92.

152. "The size of the main . . .": Wansink, B. & C. S. Wansink, "The largest Last Supper: depictions of food portions and plate size increased over the millennium," *International Journal of Obesity*, 2010, vol. 34, pp. 943–44.

152. "Here are four practical . . .": Wansink, B., *Mindless Eating: Why We Eat More Than We Think*, Bantam Books, New York, 2006.

152. "If you buy food in . . .": Marchiori, D., O. Corneille & O. Klein, "Container size influences snack food intake independently of portion size," *Appetite*, 2012, vol. 58, pp. 814–17.

153. "You might actually . . .": Shah, M., R. Schroeder & B. Adams-Huet, "A pilot study to investigate the effect of plate size on energy intake in normal weight and overweight/obese women," *Journal of Human Nutrition and Dietetics*, 2011, vol. 24, pp. 612–15.

153. "Research suggests the greater . . .": Rolls, B., E. Rowe, E. Rolls, B. Kingston, A. Megson & R. Gunary, "Variety in a meal enhances food intake in man," *Physiology and Behavior*, 1981, vol. 26, pp. 215–21; McCrory, M., P. Fuss, J. McCallum, M. Yao, A. Vinken, N. Hays & S. Roberts, "Dietary variety within food groups: association with energy intake and body fatness in men and women," *American Journal of Clinical Nutrition*, 1999, vol. 69, pp. 440–47.

153. "The bright side of . . .": McCrory, M., P. Fuss, J. McCallum, M. Yao, A. Vinken, N. Hays & S. Roberts, "Dietary variety within food groups: association with energy intake and body fatness in men and women," *American Journal of Clinical Nutrition*, 1999, vol. 69, pp. 440–47.

153. "So the trick here . . .": Raynor, H., R. Jeffery & R. Wing, "Relationship between changes in food group variety, dietary intake, and weight during obesity treatment," *International Journal of Obesity*, 2004, vol. 28, pp. 813–20.

153. "If, for example . . .": Wansink, B., "Environmental factors that increase the food intake and consumption volume of unknowing consumers," *Annual Review of Nutrition*, 2004, vol. 24, pp. 455–579.

154. "Research shows that we eat . . .": Wansink, B., "Environmental factors that increase the food intake and consumption volume of unknowing consumers," *Annual Review of*

Nutrition, 2004, vol. 24, pp. 455–579; Blass, E. M., D. R. Anderson, H. L. Kirkorian, T. A. Pempek, I. Price & M. F. Koleini, "On the road to obesity: television viewing increases intake of high-density foods," *Physiology and Behavior*, 2006, vol. 88, pp. 597–604; Stroebel, N. & J. Castro, "Listening to music while eating is related to increases in people's food intake and meal duration," *Appetite*, 2006, vol. 47, pp. 285–89; Oldham-Cooper, R., C. Hardman, C. Nicoll, P. Rogers & J. Brunstrom, "Playing a computer game during lunch affects fullness, memory for lunch, and later snack intake," *American Journal of Clinical Nutrition*, 2011, vol. 93, pp. 308–13.

154. "People tend to eat 28 . . .": de Castro, J. & M. Brewer, "The amount eaten in meals by humans is a function of the number of people present," *Physiology and Behavior*, 1991, vol. 51, no. 1, pp. 121–25.

155. "A wealth of research . . .": Wansink, B., "Environmental factors that increase the food intake and consumption volume of unknowing consumers," *Annual Review of Nutrition*, 2004, vol. 24, pp. 455–579; Chandon, P. & B. Wansink, "When are stockpiled products consumed faster? A convenience–salience framework of post-purchase consumption incidence and quantity," *Journal of Marketing Research*, 2002, vol. 39, pp. 321–25; Wansink, B., J. Painter & Y.-K. Lee, "The office candy dish: proximity's influence on estimated and actual consumption," *International Journal of Obesity*, 2006, vol. 30, pp. 871–75.

155. "People eat more chocolate . . .": Wansink, B., J. Painter & Y.-K. Lee, "The office candy dish: proximity's influence on estimated and actual consumption," *International Journal of Obesity*, 2006, vol. 30, pp. 871–75.

155. "Similarly, people tend . . .": Wansink, B., "Environmental factors that increase the food intake and consumption volume of unknowing consumers," *Annual Review of Nutrition*, 2004, vol. 24, pp. 455–579.

155. "Other research suggests . . .": Chandon, P. & B. Wansink, "When are stockpiled products consumed faster? A convenience–salience framework of post-purchase consumption incidence and quantity," *Journal of Marketing Research*, 2002, vol. 39, pp. 321–25.

CHAPTER 9: FINDING LASTING MOTIVATION

158. "This fight occurs via . . .": Rosenbaum, M. & R. Leibel, "Adaptive thermogenesis in humans," *International Journal of Obesity*, 2010, vol. 34, pp. s47–s55; Eckel, R. H., "Nonsurgical management of obesity in adults," *New England Journal of Medicine*, 2008, vol. 358, pp. 1941–50.

158. "The metabolism of people . . .": Leibel, R., M. Rosenbaum & J. Hirsch, "Changes in energy expenditure resulting from altered body weight," *New England Journal of Medicine*, 1995, vol. 332, pp. 621–28; Leibel, R. & J. Hirsch, "Diminished energy requirements in reduced-obese patients," *Metabolism*, 1983, vol. 33, pp. 164–70.

158. "Indeed, a formerly overweight . . .": Rosenbaum, M. & R. Leibel, "Adaptive thermogenesis in humans," *International Journal of Obesity*, 2010, vol. 34, pp. s47–s55.

158. "And if that isn't bad . . .": Rosenbaum, M. & R. Leibel, "Adaptive thermogenesis in humans," *International Journal of Obesity*, 2010, vol. 34, pp. s47–s55; Eckel, R. H., "Nonsurgical management of obesity in adults," *New England Journal of Medicine*, 2008, vol. 358, pp. 1941–50.

159. "Sustained weight loss is possible . . .": De Zwaan, M., A. Hilbert, S. Herpertz, S. Beutel,

O. Gefeller & B. Muelhlhans, "Weight loss maintenance in a population-based sample of German adults," *Obesity*, 2008, vol. 16, no. 11, pp. 2535–2540; McGuire, M., R. Wing & J. Hill, "The prevalence of weight loss maintenance among American adults," *International Journal of Obesity*, 1999, vol. 23, pp. 1314–1319.

159. "It turns out our body . . .": Rosenbaum, M. & R. Leibel, "Adaptive thermogenesis in humans," *International Journal of Obesity*, 2010, vol. 34, pp. s47–s55; Rosenbaum, M., J. Hirsch, D. Gallagher & R. Leibel, "Long-term persistence of adaptive thermogenesis in subjects who have maintained a reduced body weight," *American Journal of Clinical Nutrition*, 2008, vol. 88, pp. 906–12; Sumithran, P., L. Predergast, E. Delbridge, K. Purcell, A. Shuckles *et al.* "Long-term persistence of hormonal adaptations to weight loss," *New England Journal of Medicine*, 2011, vol. 17, pp. 1597–1604.

159. "Here are some statistics . . .": McGuire, M., R. Wing & J. Hill, "The prevalence of weight loss maintenance among American adults," *International Journal of Obesity*, 1999, vol. 23, pp. 1314–19.

162. "lower motivation to exercise . . .": Magnus, C. M. R., K. C. Kowalski & T. F. McHugh, "The role of self-compassion in women's self-determined motives to exercise and exercise-related outcomes," *Self and Identity*, 2010, vol. 9, pp. 363–82.

162. "lower wellbeing": Barnard, L. & J. Curry, "Self-compassion: conceptualizations, correlates, and interventions," *Review of General Psychology*, 2011, vol. 15, pp. 289–303.

162. "worse response to negative . . .": Leary, M., E. Tate, C. Adams, A. Allen & J. Hancock, "Self-compassion and reactions to unpleasant self-relevant events: the implications of treating oneself kindly," *Journal of Personality and Social Psychology*, 2007, vol. 92, pp. 887–904.

162. "worse response to failure . . .": Breines, J. & S. Chen, "Self-compassion increases self-improvement motivation," *Personality and Social Psychology Bulletin*, 2012, vol. 38, pp. 1133–43.

CHAPTER 10: SATISFYING YOUR TRUE HUNGER

171. "The first crucial step . . .": Duhigg, C., *The Power of Habit: Why We Do What We Do and How to Change*, Random House, New York, 2012.

175. "Tiredness is one . . .": McAllister, E. J., N. V. Dhurandhar, S. W. Keith *et al.*, "Ten putative contributors to the obesity epidemic," *Critical Review of Food Science and Nutrition*, 2009, vol. 49, no. 10, pp. 868–913.

175. "Indeed, sleep deprivation . . .": McAllister, E. J., N. V. Dhurandhar, S. W. Keith *et al.*, "Ten putative contributors to the obesity epidemic," *Critical Review of Food Science and Nutrition*, 2009, vol. 49, no. 10, pp. 868–913.

178. "You realize it's . . .": Tsatsoulis, A. & S. Fountoulakis, "The protective role of exercise on stress system dysregulation and comorbidities," *Annals of New York Acadamy of Sciences*, 2006, vol. 1083, pp. 196–213.

179. "If the energy . . .": Tsatsoulis, A. & S. Fountoulakis, "The protective role of exercise on stress system dysregulation and comorbidities," *Annals of New York Acadamy of Sciences*, 2006, vol. 1083, pp. 196–213.

179. "Furthermore, when we're . . .": Dallman, M., "Stress-induced obesity and the emotional nervous system," *Trends in Endocrinology and Metabolism*, 2010, vol. 21, pp. 159–65.

179. "Probably the single . . .": Tsatsoulis, A. & S. Fountoulakis, "The protective role of exercise on stress system dysregulation and comorbidities," *Annals of New York Acadamy of Sciences*, 2006, vol. 1083, pp. 196–213.

179. "It could be something . . .": Thayer, R., "Energy, tiredness and tension effects of a sugar snack versus moderate exercise," *Journal of Personality and Social Psychology*, 1987, vol. 52, no. 1, pp. 119–129.

180. "Another scientifically supported . . .": Sedlmeier, P., J. Eberth, M. Schwarz, D. Zimmermann & F. Haarig, "The psychological effects of meditation: a meta-analysis," *Psychological Bulletin*, 2012, pp. 1–33.

180. "Again, we don't have to . . .": Arch, J. J., & M. G. Craske, "Mechanisms of mindfulness: emotion regulation following a focused breathing induction," *Behavior Research and Therapy, 2006, vol. 44*, no. 12, pp. 1849–58.

Broderick, P. C., "Mindfulness and coping with dysphoric mood: contrasts with rumination and distraction," *Cognitive Therapy and Research,* 2005, vol. 29, no. 5, pp. 501–510; W. L. Heppner, M. H. Kernis, C. E. Lakey, W. K. Campbell, B. M. Goldman, P. J. Davis, and E. V. Cascio, "Mindfulness as a means of reducing aggressive behavior: dispositional and situational evidence," *Aggressive Behavior,* 2008, vol. 34, no. 5, pp. 486–96; Sanders, W. & D. H. Lam, "Ruminative and mindful self-focused processing modes and their impact on problem solving in dysphoric individuals," *Behavior Research and Therapy,* 2010, vol. 48, no. 8, pp. 747–53.

CHAPTER 11: ENHANCE YOUR LIFE

187. "When we're cut . . .": Diener, E. & M. Seligman, "Very happy people," *Psychological Science*, 2002, vol. 13, no. 1, pp. 81–84; Uchino, B., "Understanding the links between social support and physical health," *Perspectives on Psychological Science*, 2009, vol. 4, pp. 236–55.

187. "Research suggests that . . .": Csikszentmihalyi, M. & J. Hunter, "Happiness in everday life: the uses of experience sampling," *Journal of Happiness Studies*, 2003, vol. 4, pp. 185–99.

187. "The most fulfilled people . . .": Myers, D. G., *The Pursuit of Happiness: Who Is Happy and Why*, William Morrow, New York, 1992; Csikszentmihalyi, M. & M. M.-H. Wong, "The situational and personal correlates of happiness: a cross-national comparison," in F. Strack, M. Argyle & N. Schwarz (eds), *Subjective Well-being: An Interdisciplinary Perspective*, Pergamon Press, Oxford, 1991, pp. 193–212.

188. "In this state . . .": Csikszentmihalyi, M., "The flow experience and its significance for human psychology," in M. Csikszentmihalyi & I. S. Csikszentmihalyi (eds), *Optimal Experience: Psychological Studies of Flow in Consciousness*, Cambridge University Press, Cambridge, 1988, pp. 15–35; Csikszentmihalyi, M., *Finding Flow: The Psychology of Engagement with Everyday Life*, Basic Books, New York, 1997.

188. "The flow experience . . .": Csikszentmihalyi, M., *Finding Flow: The Psychology of*

Engagement with Everyday Life, Basic Books, New York, 1997.

188. "Nevertheless, the average . . .": Csikszentmihalyi, M., *Finding Flow: The Psychology of Engagement with Everyday Life*, Basic Books, New York, 1997.

189. "We like to be . . .": Deci, E. L., "Effects of externally mediated rewards on instrinsic motivation," *Journal of Personality and Social Psychology*, 1971, vol. 18, pp. 105–15; Brown, N., D. Read & B. Summers, "The lure of choice," *Journal of Behavioral Decision Making*, 2003, vol. 16, pp. 297–308.

189. "If you get paid . . .": Deci, E. L., "Effects of externally mediated rewards on instrinsic motivation," *Journal of Personality and Social Psychology*, 1971, vol. 18, pp. 105–15; Brown, N., D. Read & B. Summers, "The lure of choice," *Journal of Behavioral Decision Making*, 2003, vol. 16, pp. 297–308.

189. "In general, more . . .": Myers, D. G., *The Pursuit of Happiness: Who Is Happy and Why*, William Morrow, New York, 1992.

CHAPTER 12: FINDING YOUR FAITH AND COURAGE

196. "Another important feature . . .": Logel, C. & G. Cohen, "The role of the self in physical health: testing the effect of a values-affirmation intervention on weight loss," *Psychological Science*, 2012, vol. 23, pp. 53–55.

RESOURCES

For free resources related to this book, further information regarding ACT, and details of workshops and training, please visit:
theweightescape.com

You may also wish to visit:
actmindfully.com.au
actforadolescents.com

ACKNOWLEDGMENTS

We would like to acknowledge all the hard working and supportive people at Penguin who made this possible, including Daniel Hudspith and Andrea McNamara. We would also like to acknowledge our mentors—Steve Hayes, Kelly Wilson, Kirk Stroshal, and the broader ACT community.

INDEX

ABOUT THE AUTHORS

Dr Joseph Ciarrochi is Professor of Psychology at the University of Western Sydney and a renowned ACT trainer and researcher. Joseph has published over ninety papers, books and book chapters. In 2011, he won a prestigious Australian Research Council Future Fellow award, which recognizes him as one of the top scientists in the Australia. He is, along with Ann Bailey, one of the authors of the bestselling self-help book, *Get Out of Your Mind and Into Your Life for Teens*.

Ann Bailey, MA, Senior Clinical Psychologist, has designed and implemented an award-winning government service. She is currently the psychological consultant for dieticians in South Eastern Sydney Illawarra Health, running workshops and coaching allied health staff on the principles of ACT for health and well-being. Ann has been featured in the influential ACT in Action video training series as a master clinician and is the coauthor of a number of ACT books.

Dr Russ Harris qualified as a doctor in the UK before emigrating to Australia in 1991. He now works as a therapist and executive coach, as well as being an internationally acclaimed ACT trainer. He is the bestselling author of seven books, including *The Reality Slap*, *The Confidence Gap*, and his best-known work, *The Happiness Trap*, which has now been translated into thirty different languages.

theweightescape.com